Fighting For Allergy-Free Food: The
Extended Interviews

First Printing: 2017

ISBN 978-1-387-10898-5

Captain Purple Productions, LLC

www.FightingForAllergyFreeFood.com

www.CaptainPurpleProductions.com

TABLE OF CONTENTS

INTRODUCTION

I spent over a year traveling and interviewing the best people I could find to ask the same questions: Why are there so many food allergies, sensitivities and intolerances? Where do they come from? Where is this heading? And that led to many more questions instead of answers. What is genetically modified food? Why are we making genetically modified food? What's the government doing to protect us? Etcetera. I went into this with an open mind, going after interviews that could present both sides to every question. These interviews turned into the feature documentary, *Fighting For Allergy-Free Food*.

What follows are selected extended transcripts of every interview I did. They've been edited for clarity and content, with no paraphrasing and hopefully without at all changing the meaning behind what people said. Please realize these were conversations, and they read that way. Some people have accents or speech patterns that are more challenging to read, and I've again tried to just edit it enough to make it easier for clarity.

Thank you to everyone that allowed me to interview them.

Thank you for reading. Keep fighting for allergy-free food.

Tamar Kummel, filmmaker

Gene: I'm Gene Stollerman. I'm an emeritus professor of Boston University. And I've been professor of medicine at the University of Tennessee and Northwestern University, New York University, and then Columbia University.

Anything that I had to do that involved relief of human suffering was going to be all right with me. But the area that attracted most of my attention throughout my career was inflammation. And everybody said, "Well that's everything." Yeah I said, that's your reaction to injury. The body's reaction to injury is what we know of as inflammation.

And one of the most difficult things we have to do in medicine is sort out the different things that cause inflammation, because they're all interrelated. And therefore, we give names to things sometimes that are inappropriate. After you know more about them, they no longer apply. So changing the name often is because we know more and more about them. Right?

Now let me tell you that the most difficult to explain is "allergy." You're not reacting like you should. You're allergic. Right? Now where'd this come from? It came really at the dawn of the 20th century. At the beginning of the 20th century was the beginning of the whole field of what we call now, immunology. Immunology is a study of a defense of an individual against anything that threatens the individual from infection to trauma. Anything that's assaultive can be considered.

[5]

But allergy got its name when we were beginning to learn there were such things as antibodies. Antibodies then were discovered at the beginning of the 19th century, mainly from toxins like diphtheria. When diphtheria's toxins were made, it was found, if you add an antibody to it you can inject an animal with a toxin and he would then become immune to the disease by having an antibody develop against a toxin. We began to find out that when we began studying antibodies, they were not all benign. That is, if you gave an antibody to somebody that would prevent the disease, that person may get sick.

The problem with "allergy" as a name, is that almost everybody can have an antibody to something that makes them allergic to it-- which means they get a reaction to it when they eat it, or when they smell it, or when they feel it, touch it. All those things can make you break out in a rash, run a fever, have an upset stomach. So those are reactions that you have that are protecting you against foreign materials.

Now, why don't we all get a reaction to it? Well, there are some people that make an excess of what we call IgE. That is the antibody that is causing vaccine-allergic reactions. The IgE is an antibody that is in itself causing reaction when you make too much of it. So you shouldn't make an excess of IgE. It's there to help you, but some people are genetically disposed. Families have a very high incidence of allergy within the family. Twins... about 80% of twins will be allergic to the same thing. So, we have a whole field that's been developed that deals with that group of diseases that depend on abnormal antibodies. And that's what the allergists usually do. But immunology is much bigger than that.

And one area that's really mystified us is food allergy. I said that you recognize any compound that's not you. Well, what happens when you eat all these things that you're eating? You eat every kind of food that's got every kind of chemical, why don't you make antibodies to everything? And the answer is because you're made to recognize things that are harmful, but not necessarily good things. So, if you say you have an allergy to milk, the truth is, you don't have an allergy to milk. Milk is one of the things, you have an *intolerance*, because you don't have enough lactic enzyme that digests lactic acid. So that is not an allergy; that's a food intolerance for a different reason. But for years it was called food allergy. And a lot of things are called food allergy that may not be food allergy. They may be what we call intolerance.

Now how do you know what's tolerant or not? Unfortunately, it's the most complicated area yet. The area that decides what you can eat and what you can't, is laid down in the first few months of your life. But it's the most complicated part of immunology-- to learn how we can be tolerant to most foods and react to other foods.

Let's look for example at gluten. For a long time, we called that disease a sprue-like disease. You had a certain disease and you had a fatty diarrhea and terrible loss of weight. And we called it sprue. And we only knew you could eat certain things. Gradually it dawned on people that there were some foods that, like wheat, that were particularly bad. And when they

[7]

began to study it they found there was a protein called gluten that was in wheat, but a lot of other, too, that you were particularly liable to become intolerant to, or to be intolerant. And that was a genetic thing, also. It was, people didn't have whatever you need to protect you against a reaction to gluten. They're lacking a protection. And that's what we know about gluten enteropathy. It has enabled people to get along that used to have a terrible time.

Now with regard to other things, there were people, for example, who really are allergic to peanut oil-- to the protein in peanuts, the protein, not the oil. The protein in the peanut is extremely able to make IGE. And for people who make a lot of IGE, the frequency is very great of having peanut allergy. And that's a real allergy. That could be so acute that smelling a peanut can give you a rash.

Tamar: Food allergies and intolerances are definitely increasing. But do you think that we have always been intolerant, or that there's suddenly a new proliferation of food allergies and why?

Gene: Questions like that are extremely hard to answer epidemiologically for several reasons. The more a subject becomes studied, the more people become aware of it. And the more people are aware of it, the more they look to see if they have it. So people never heard of a certain disease. Once they hear it's in the family they'll be looking for it and they'll be sure probably, in most cases, to find it.

So the problem of finding the unknown case is one of the big subjects of the epidemiology, we call it, of allergy. The other thing is that we have had a tremendous increase in prepared foods. The number of prepared foods is huge. And every one of those foods uses a huge amount of some flour. They may use potato flour, they may use wheat flour, corn flour. But you can be sure that almost every food is going to have a lot of different things in it. And those foods may become popular. And the more you eat them, the more people you can discover can have reactions to them.

Peanuts are a good example. Peanuts was one of the things we learned most about because it was so spectacular-- as a cause of classical allergy. And looking at the question, "Is peanut allergy increasing or not," would be a lot easier than looking at something that was much more difficult to study. Peanut, you have a clear antigen, you know the antibody, you know how to study it. You have all those factors.

Dr. Stollerman's career in research, education and patient care includes his involvement in the great medical advances of the past century, particularly the eradication of rheumatic heart disease in developed countries, and currently the creation of a vaccine against the cause of rheumatic fever, streptococcal sore throat, for developing countries. (Amazon.com)

Dr. Stollerman passed away 8/1/2014

Whitney Morgan Block, MSN, CPNP, FNP-BC
Interviewed 2/13/15

Tamar: OK. Just to start off, tell me about yourself, where you work, the lab, just tell me everything.

Whitney: So I am a pediatric nurse practitioner, a clinical research nurse practitioner. I grew up in Atlanta, Georgia, and then I went to school in Johns Hopkins in Baltimore. Went through an accelerated BSN program. Then got my Masters at Vanderbilt University.

So right now we are at El Camino hospital in Mountain View, California. I technically work for Stanford School of Medicine, and they run a food allergy center. Just recently we got renamed and rebranded to the Sean N. Parker Center for Allergy Research, which we're really excited about.

So, what we pretty much do here is a little bit different then what we do in outpatient land. What we do here is specifically food allergy research. So we're running right now about 11 different clinical trials. And we see kids that are severely, severely allergic. So we're actually going through a screening process right now to fill up some of our new upcoming trials.

What we're kind of known for here in Stanford is the multiple food allergy research that we do-- so desensitizing to multiple foods at the same time, which has never really been done anywhere in the world. So people come from all over the world to get this amazing treatment. They call it treatment. We still consider it research because it's not out there to the public. However, that's kind of our goal that we're striving towards. We're hoping that eventually we can find out the secret recipe, the exact science behind it, what exactly we should do so people can learn about it in nursing schools.

And you don't have to come here to Mountain View, California to get this awesome treatment, and to potentially, eventually get cured of your allergies. We don't call it a cure yet because we don't know exactly the long-term benefits of it. But what we're hoping for is that anybody from middle-country Nebraska to all the way where I'm originally from in Atlanta, Georgia, everybody would be able to have access to this awesome treatment to be able to manage their food allergies.

So that's really what we're doing around here. The screening process is pretty long, kind of hard for a lot of these families. We've got over 1,000 people on our waiting list right now. And they contacted us up to 2 and 3 years ago interested in our research.

Tamar: Do you think that food allergies are more prevalent now or that we're more able to diagnose that now?

Whitney: Food allergies are definitely more prevalent. The CDC came out in 2013 and said that food allergies have increased 50% between 1987 and 2011. So they're definitely more prevalent today.

Tamar: And why do you think that is?

Whitney: We really don't know. There are a lot of theories out there. But I wouldn't be able to exactly say. I think that it's probably a mixture between nature and nurture, meaning that there's something in the genetics. But there's definitely an environmental component as well. And it's how those two interplay that determines whether you have a food allergy or not.

Tamar: So, talk to me about food allergies.

Whitney: With a food allergy, it doesn't depend on the amount of the food. It doesn't depend on what type of food it is. It's every single time you get exposed to that protein that your threshold is set off. You're going to get that chemical reaction. You're going to get an allergic reaction from it.

Tamar: And would you elaborate on what part the FDA actually has on making sure our food is safe?

Whitney: So, I know that other countries kind of do it better than we do, and so there's definitely room for improvement in my mind as to what our government could be doing. The FDA does play a very big role in all of our research because since we're giving all of these foods in all of our trials as to elicit a response, the government looks at it as we're giving a drug. So they actually have to approve every single food that we give in all of our trials. And so that's kind of one of the hurdles later on with, when or if this actually becomes approved for the general population and so your local allergist would be able to do immunotherapy. The question is, who's going to pay for it, who's going to sponsor it-- and those kinds of things.

And that's where we're going to have a lot of discussions, I think, with the government coming up about should we consider this a food? Should we consider this a drug? How much oversight do we need in this process when it gets out to the general population? Are you actually going to have to go to a pharmacy and pick up your peanut prescription? Or is it going to be something that you can just sell over the counter. So there's a lot that's going to go into it. We don't know how it's going to end.

Whitney Morgan Block, MSN, CPNP, FNP-BC
Sean N. Parker Center for Allergy Research at Stanford University
Stanford University School of Medicine

Tamar: So just say your name.

Brandy: Hi. I'm Brandy Wendler. I have Celiac disease.

Tamar: Okay. So tell me a little about how you figured that out. How your journey's been.

Brandy: I was diagnosed 6 years ago. It was about 10 years where I had symptoms, gastrointestinal symptoms. I had always struggled with the neurological issues like anxiety, depression, different things like that, just, brain fog. And I always struggled with those during high school, but we kind of just figured that was the way that I am. And the gastrointestinal symptoms, I just figured that I had a lot of fiber in my diet. I didn't really understand.

We didn't put two and two together until my thyroid started failing. And it wasn't until I developed Hashimoto's thyroiditis, which is very common in those with untreated Celiac disease-- they typically develop a secondary autoimmune disease if it goes untreated for a long time-- that I was diagnosed with Celiac disease. And when I was diagnosed, I was a nurse in a cardiovascular ICU. I was getting my master's. And I had had several colleagues who looked at my symptoms, looked at my lab work, talked to me, of course, about my life and said, "nothing's wrong, you're stressed out, you work night shift, you're probably just tired." Even though I was sleeping 16, 18 hours a day. Still never feeling fully rested. I was anxious all the time. I was getting

[14]

married and I was still depressed and crying a lot. And I wasn't really living a quality life. I was living-- I wasn't really living. I was more *suffering* through life.

So when I was diagnosed, I thought to myself, "How many people like me don't get diagnosed?" I'm in the medical field and I didn't get the help I needed. So how many people without medical training don't get the help that they need? So, that's kind of how I started down this journey of raising awareness and traveling and speaking about Celiac disease.

Tamar: Where/who was the first person that said, "Hey, let's test you?"

Brandy: That's actually interesting. I saw over a dozen different physicians from different specialties. I saw a rheumatoid physician because I used to have bilateral swelling in my fingers and knees and hips. And I had an elevated sedimentation rate. I saw a neurologist for my depression. They thought I had MS because I had some weird issues going on with my muscles, and so I saw a bunch of general practitioners, I saw an endocrinologist, and finally, I saw an OBYGYN that tested me for everything under the sun, realized that my cortisol levels were off and that my thyroids had been trending down. And no one had ever done a full thyroid panel, so he did. And it was very interesting to see what he found. And my cortisol levels had been trending down. And he said, "I really don't know what to do for you." He said, "I can treat this, but you have other issues and I can't figure it out, so go see this guy," which was another endocrinologist, who actually had Celiac disease himself.

So when he saw me he said, "You have Hashimoto's thyroiditis." I said, "I know! I have thyroid disease. I've been screaming that at the top of my lungs." And he said, "But you also have Celiac disease." And I was like, (LAUGH) "nobody has Celiac disease, it's so rare." And he was like, "No, you have it." And we argued back and forth and I went gluten free for two weeks, didn't think I noticed a difference until I actually had-- it was the 4th of July, I decided I was going to quit this whole gluten-free thing and have a hot dog-- and I vomited the whole rest of the evening and felt horrible. So then, you know, I said, "Oh, maybe's he's got a little something to him. Maybe he knows a thing or two." And my blood tests were positive. I have both the DQ2 and DQ8 genes for Celiac disease. So I have Celiac disease, despite my denial at the beginning.

Tamar: Any other food allergies?

Brandy: I cannot do cow's milk. I have an allergy to casein and soy. I actually will react to those 2 faster than I will to gluten. I guess because gluten is more immune in me and kills off the villi in my small intestine. But I think because I was undiagnosed for so long, my system started to cross-react to those two because the protein sizes, in casein in particular, are very similar to gliadin, and the soy protein is so much larger that I can't have either of those without my having a gut reaction-- different symptoms based on the food, but still a gut reaction. A lot of people can add back in dairy after they've gone gluten free for six months, a year, two years. I waited two-and-a-half years, tried to add back in dairy and my thyroid levels went crazy. So I can't do either of them. Soy, I would never go back to because I get such bad stomach pains. But dairy, sometimes I just want some cheese or something. And I can't go back to either of those. So I avoid them.

Tamar: Do you think that food allergies are more prevalent now, or do you think we're more able to diagnose it now?

Brandy: I think we're more aware of them now. However, they have doubled in the past 10 years. Especially in children, you've gone from about 3% of children having food allergies to over 5% of children having allergies. And the same is with adults. The rate has doubled-- and the prevalence. The knowledge in the community has increased as well.

Tamar: So why do you think that is?

Brandy: There are several theories for that. One of my favorites is the hygiene theory, meaning that we as a society is cleaner in our daily habits and so our gut isn't exposed to the same microbes that it used to be. You have lots of studies to support that children that grow up in the country have better immune systems than children that grow up in the city. So I think that plays a part.

I also think that our processed foods play a part. People in our society-- peanuts for example-- we tend to roast peanuts. And we have high peanut allergies. But in other countries, where roasting is not a normal process of serving peanuts, they boil them. They don't have as many peanut allergies. So part of processing can play a part in that.

I also think genetically modified foods play a part in that. Because our bodies may not necessarily recognize them. And we've gone from having a variety to having one or two that are "stronger strains" that are genetically modified. And then you have some more minor theories, too, that I think may also play a role, like the antioxidant theory, whereas we're eating more processed, more packaged fruits and vegetables and we're not getting fresh, raw fruits and vegetables. The antioxidants just help in processing the food and help get rid of any proteins that are bad that your stomach may absorb. So there's that theory.

And then there's also a dietary fat theory, meaning that we get more vegetable fats instead of animal fats and things that our bodies weren't originally created to deal with. So I don't necessarily think that it's just one thing. I think it's multifactorial. You may have a couple of those things going on at one time.

Tamar: So what do you think about the current trend in people avoiding gluten, even if they're not intolerant?

Brandy: I think there are pros and cons to that. When I was gluten free, when I first started being gluten free even six years ago, there wasn't a lot of availability of products. But now that it's become, "the fad," there's a lot of things that are available, and restaurants are starting to have gluten-free menus and they're starting to be conscious about that in their customers. And even the price of gluten-free food has decreased a little bit because it's becoming so popular.

You have, not all gluten-free food, but you have some companies like Pillsbury who's doing gluten-free dough and gluten-free cookie dough and things like that. And that can be found at fair prices. I know at the BX on base I can get it for $2.50. So that's pretty exciting. So you have those pros of it. But the cons of it tend to be that a lot of people will say they're gluten free even though it's more of a preference in eating instead of someone like me who has to have that.

And so there's some confusion in the community about that. And then you run the risk of being taken not as seriously when you say, "Oh, I can't do gluten," because you have people who are like, "Oh, I can't do it, but I'm gonna eat this little bite of something." And so there are a lot of people like, "Oh, you can just pick the croutons off." I'm like, "No, that's not how it works with me. That may be great for your diet and losing weight, but that's not how it works for me." So you have pros and cons of both sides. If you focus on the good things, then we're OK.

Tamar: All right. What do you think it would surprise us to learn? Is there anything else? Anything that you want to talk about personally?

Brandy: That I want to talk about? I think Celiac disease eventually will-- gluten intolerances in general will-- become almost a spectrum, like autism. I think you'll have your Celiac disease, your gluten intolerance, gluten allergies, and they'll discover more of that. I'm actually kind of looking forward to it.

But like I said earlier, I really think our convenience is killing us. What seems easy and fast at the moment is not what's good for us. Even foods that cause just inflammation-- not necessarily an allergy, not necessarily an intolerance-- but they're highly inflammatory in the body, like sugar-- or, you know, we have way too much GMO corn, dairy and gluten.

Vanessa: I'm Vanessa Weisbrod and I'm the executive director of *Delight Gluten-Free Magazine* and I also sit on the board of directors of the Celiac Disease program at Children's National Medical Center.

Tamar: What's your personal story?

Vanessa: So, when I was a little kid, I was diagnosed with every allergy on the block. I couldn't have milk, eggs, strawberries, oranges, lettuce. So many things they said I was allergic to. And the strange thing was, gluten was never one of those things that doctors suggested I was allergic to. Strangely enough, when I finally got diagnosed with Celiac Disease, I was about 21, so about 10 years ago. Once I went gluten free, every single allergy they said I had, completely went away. So now I can eat all those things they said I couldn't have.

Tamar: What is the number one allergy that you feel is starting to come up even more?

Vanessa: Dairy. Everyone is dairy. There's a handful of people who say they have corn issues. We get a lot of potato calls, too.

Tamar: What do you think it would surprise us to learn?

Vanessa: That you don't know how crappy you're feeling until you take gluten out of your diet. That it's really eye-opening. I never had stomach aches until about six months before I was diagnosed. Since I was an infant, I had seizures and horrible migraine headaches. Saw every neurologist. I grew up in California in San Francisco. They were always like, "Yeah, she just has really bad migraine headaches," like, "She has seizures, not really sure, hopefully she'll out grow them." Tried every medication. Nothing helped. Goodness knows how much I poisoned myself with different drugs. And within two weeks of going gluten free, I woke-- I just remember the first day I woke up and I didn't feel like there was this dark cloud of just not feeling-- well, hanging over my head. And I was like, "Really?! Because I was eating wheat?!" It's just so mind-boggling that something so basic and so simple can cause so many health problems for people.

Vanessa Maltin Weisbrod is the Executive Editor of *Delight Gluten-Free Magazine*, an international publication geared towards people with food allergies, Celiac disease and other medical conditions relating to food. In addition to the magazine, Vanessa also consults for a variety of gluten-free food manufactures and is an active member of the Advisory Board of the Celiac Disease Center at Children's National Medical Center.

Vanessa is also the author of two gluten-free cookbooks: *Beyond Rice Cakes: A Young Person's Guide to Cooking, Eating & Living Gluten-Free* was released in September 2006 and her second book is *The Gloriously Gluten-Free Cookbook: Spicing Up Life with Italian, Asian and Mexican Recipes* (Wiley) was released in April 2010.

Vanessa has appeared on numerous television shows as a gluten-free food and Celiac disease expert including Planet Green's *Emeril Green*, CNBC's *On The Money* and CNN's *Newsroom with Heidi Collins*. She has been interviewed and quoted in *U.S. News & World Report*,

Newsweek, The Washington Post, Washington Woman, Supermarket News, Publix *Greenwise Magazine* and numerous other local newspapers.

Vanessa received a bachelor's degree in journalism from the George Washington University and a Culinary Arts degree from the Institute of Culinary Education. She also holds certificates in the Practical Applications of Food Allergy Guidelines and Nutritional Analysis for Federal School Breakfast & Lunch Programs. Previously she worked as a health care reporter for the Advisory Board Company's Daily Briefing and for Cox Newspapers, where she covered healthcare, politics, immigration and other breaking news for major newspapers including the *Palm Beach Post,* the *Atlanta Journal-Constitution,* and the *Dayton Daily News.* (gfafexpo.com)

George: So food allergies and sensitivities and intolerance are really all related to food but they're very different things. Allergies are a type of hypersensitivity reaction that's mediated by a certain part of the immune system called IgE, Immunoglobulin E. And you have an immediate, within 20-minute reaction-- allergic reaction-- where your body produces certain chemicals-- you know, the typical your throat closes, your lips blow up, etcetera, food allergy.

Food sensitivity is also an immune issue, but it's not a hypersensitivity issue and it's mediated by something called IgG or Immunoglobulin G, different part of the immune system. And it's a delayed reaction. It could be up to four days. And it creates symptoms that aren't always gastrointestinal. Those symptoms can be joint pain or gas or headache or many other types of things like that.

An intolerance is not an immune mediated thing. For instance, lactose intolerance, or you eat beans and it causes gas, or you eat this kind of food and it makes your tongue tingle. Those are reactions that you have to something where you're intolerant to it, but it's not a disease.

Tamar: It's very common, though, for there to be similar symptoms or confusing symptoms where some people will get several different reactions to the same food or several foods at the same time?

George: So they're each really independent of each other. But you can be allergic to wheat and sensitive to wheat. Right? You can have both. So yes, people can have both-- or all three-- in theory.

Tamar: Do you think food allergies are more prevalent now? Or do you think that we're more able to diagnose it now?

George: Well I think both are true. Our diagnostic testing is definitely getting better. And there are certain labs that are really very good at it. But not yet the national labs. Not the routine labs that most physicians use. They're very limited in that. But I think the prevalence also is getting better as our food system changes. As we genetically change because of these issues, we pass those genes on to our children. So it is getting more prevalent also.

Tamar: Is there good testing now for Celiac or do we still not have a conclusive test?

George: Well, if you want to know if you have Celiac disease, right now, the standard for diagnosis is a biopsy, where you look to see if you have flattened villi or not. But there are blood tests and there's something called a Celiac panel, and all labs do it. It's three or four antibody tests and they can show whether you're having an immune response to gluten. Right? It's an IGG test, not an IGE test. All labs do it. But they limit it to very specific certain antibodies. As an example, Baylor University started a test where they do it in the stool, which it seems to me is more accurate than the blood. But not every state allows you to do that test. And now there's a lab called Cyrex that is doing a very, very sophisticated test, where they measure 10 or 20 different types of gluten reactions. And that's probably the up-and-coming-way to do it, but not every state will allow you to do that either.

Tamar: Why is that?

George: Well, there's been battle between mainstream medicine and complementary or alternative medicine. And mainstream medicine would like to eliminate certain of the competitions. Pharmaceutical companies would like to force you to use certain of their products as opposed to other things. That's why I think it's happening. The rationalization used is that those IgG things, or food intolerances, don't represent a disease, so we shouldn't test for them.

Tamar: So do you think this is going to keep getting worse?

George: No question. I think it's going to be getting worse for several reasons. The more we genetically modify food, the more it becomes foreign to us. And genetically modified food is really a pretty big thing now-- not just in our country, but in the world. And the second thing is, as we use pesticides and food additives and preservatives and things, those things get much further away from real food and further away from our immune system recognizing them.

And, of course, there's the issue of infections and food handlers and toxins and things that are in our food. You know, you use dirty water to water your vegetables, you eat that vegetable, you eat those toxins. And so I *do* think it's going to be an increasingly bad epidemic.

Unfortunately, we're pretty shortsighted. We would like to spend less money now and we'll worry about tomorrow, tomorrow. And as long as we do that, as long as we put antibiotics in our foods, as long as we put pesticides in our plants and preservatives in our foods, we're going to be experiencing this.

You know the food we eat today, is very different than what we ate 1,000 years ago, 100 years ago. You know everything cavemen ate was organic-- free range and organic. And even our grandparents, they went out and they picked their food. They had what they had on their farm or what their neighbors grew. They ate the way we talk now is special, "farm to table"-- you know, buy within 100 miles and sustainable. And that's an up-and-coming thing. And it's a very good thing. And it really would make a big difference.

But above that, we have to take the chemicals out of the air and out of the water. We have to take the chemicals off of the food. You know, the best example-- a good example that I can think of-- is something simple like blueberries. So blueberries, you've grown them on the farm and the farmers have made them a certain color, and a certain size, and they make them slow to deteriorate. And they create a shell that's a little thicker, so in the movement, it doesn't bruise. And they make them resistant to bugs and birds and thises and thats. And they feed them a certain way. And we get those blueberries in a store and they don't really taste so great, but they look great. But they're really different. When you get wild blueberries from the coast of Maine, which you're very familiar with, they're completely stressed out. They're frozen at night. They have salt water on them. The birds are picking at them. The insects are eating them. Those are stressed-out plants. When we eat them, first of all, they're delicious. But they contain all of these chemicals that help us. So those chemicals that the plant needs to survive, help us. And so those micronutrients are wonderful. And a lot of the food we eat looks great, but it lacks those things.

Tamar: Amazing. What do you think of the current trend of people avoiding gluten, even if they're not intolerant?

George: So, there is definitely validity to avoiding gluten. So, putting aside that we probably don't have adequate testing and that we miss a lot, probably 3% of our population is really Celiac-positive, genetically and biopsy, 2% to 3% anyway. Probably 10% are gluten sensitive by diagnosis of lab testing. But I think the population is even bigger that truly are gluten sensitive.

So, when you look at this genetically modified thing again, you're asking your body to recognize-- to process a protein that is foreign to it. So gluten, in the scheme of genetics, is about 100 years old. And you know, we're five, 10,000 years old. So, in that 100 years, in general, we have not yet found a way to process this. So many, many people have immune responses to it.

Tamar: So what do you think it would surprise us to learn? Is there anything you wanted to talk about?

George: So, the gut contains up to 80% of our total body's immune system. So that's a pretty big deal. And in that gut, we have these normal and abnormal bacteria. And they have to live harmoniously together to process food and to recognize a difference between what we would consider "me" and "not me." Right? So the body likes "me" inside of it. It doesn't like "not me" inside of it.

And when we eat food that is either not processed well, because it's poorly digested, or contains chemicals, or genetically modified, or has toxins or infections or that type of a thing, or we just lack digestive enzymes and don't process it well, our body looks at that as, "not me," and makes antibodies against what it looks like as a foreign antigen. So when you look at things like the increase in the amount of autoimmune disease-- multiple sclerosis, and lupus, and rheumatoid arthritis, and psoriasis, and those types of illnesses-- we know that a large part of that is related to gut function. And a large part of *that* is related to how we process or don't process certain foods, or the contaminants in foods.

And it turns out to be an extremely important thing in terms of the national economy, how much we spend to look at this type of illness, how much we spend to treat people who are not well, and how much it costs us personally not to feel good. And so I think that it's really a major issue for our well-being to deal with this.

What we didn't talk about, was antibiotics.

Tamar: Go for it.

George: Okay. So in that same vein are the things that we should know. We use a lot of antibiotics in our society and we're trying to get away from it-- not just because of the resistance issues where they stop working and we're going to run out of them, but even in pediatrics, where 10 years ago every time a child had an ear infection, we gave them an antibiotic.

So we know that in childhood, antibiotics kill normal bacteria. And it doesn't just kill it for that moment and, "Oh, I'll take a probiotic," and it goes away. It doesn't really work that way. We know, for instance, in the Spring of 2012 there was a study published in the *Journal of the American Medical Association* where they looked at the total number of days that a woman, by the time she was 20-something, the total number of days she took antibiotics. When it reaches a certain threshold, the incidence of breast cancer went up. And the reason that the incidence of breast cancer went up, they postulated, was that it killed your normal bacteria, and they don't grow back, and that's your immune system. And so you couldn't defend the environment. And they believe 70 or 75% of breast cancer is environmental. And so you say, "Well, I'll just give people probiotics." But it doesn't work. Because the antibiotics destroy this balance of what we call a microbiome. So there are 10 times more bacterial cells than cells in our body. We have 10 times more foreign DNA living in us than our own. And how they balance each other is how healthy we are.

These bacteria make your neurotransmitters. They make vitamins for you. They process. They send information. They're vitally important. This is really modern-day science, you know. State-of-the-art research is telling you what I'm saying now. And we've destroyed that. When you look at these people who've taken antibiotics over and over and over again and the rate of autoimmune illness and that type of thing, it's really scary.

Tamar: Are you worried about the antibiotics in all the livestock?

George: Well, I don't eat anything that comes with antibiotics in it. I think it really is an issue. We have at our grand rounds, at my hospital, repeatedly been told that we're going to run out of effective antibiotics. And we're going to have diseases that are going to be untreatable. And this is part of the reason that we've become resistant to antibiotics-- that the *bugs* become resistant to antibiotics.

Tamar: How often do you see patients that you say, "We really need to test you for food reactions"?

George: All right. Well, I would do it all the time in people who had any type of autoimmune illness. In people who have certain symptoms and have gone through repeated workups by good physicians and are told over and over, "You don't have a disease. There's nothing wrong with you. It's in your head. Take an antidepressant," I think looking for food is very important.

One problem we have is September 2013 New York State stopped us from being able to do that test. So it can't be done in New York State now.

Tamar: Can you send it out somewhere else?

George: You have to have a physician with a license from another state process the blood or the labs, or the testing, and submit it from that state.

Tamar: What are the main foods people react to?

George: It's a great question. The number one most common food sensitivity is milk and dairy products. Heads and tails above everything else. And I think the next most common, as a group, are eggs, soy, corn and gluten. But milk, far and away is the biggest. Other than cats, we're the only species of animals that drinks milk of other animals. And we're the only species where adults drink milk at all. So it's really very foreign to us. And it's not lactose intolerance, although that really is a real issue and significant. It's that we don't break down the casein-- the protein in the milk-- and have immune responses to it.

Dr. Kessler graduated from the A.T. Still University of Health Sciences/ Kirksville College of Osteopathic Medicine in 1973. He works in New York, NY and specializes in Family Medicine. Dr. Kessler is affiliated with New York Presbyterian Westchester Division. (http://doctor.webmd.com)

Tamar: What is the ADA Gluten Intolerance
Workgroup?

Anne: The Gluten Intolerance Workgroup is a group
of expert dieticians, and we were called together
years ago to start looking at the research and the
evidence on the use of the gluten-free diet in Celiac
disease and then eventually gluten sensitivity or
gluten intolerance. The reason we were pulled
together was the American Dietetic Association,
which now has been renamed to the Academy of
Nutrition and Dietetics, wanted to make sure that
experts in the field looked at the research and came
up with a plan and guidance for all dieticians to use in
treatment of Celiac disease and gluten sensitivity. The
reason being, as you said in your path, trying to find
out what to eat, what not to eat. There's a lot of
information that conflicted. So we worked together,
went through the research. It was an evidence
analysis process. So we looked at the research, rated
it, analyzed it, included those studies that met the
inclusion criteria. From there, formulated the guidance
for a gluten-free diet and then developed a tool kit that
dieticians could use. So it had the right questions to
ask on a consultation, the proper education materials
to give. So it really gave dieticians across the nation
and Canada the tools to really inform their patients,
based on evidence and scientific research, rather
than just hearsay.

Tamar: Can you explain a little bit about the cross-contamination of the normal gluten-free grains?

Anne: Yes. The study that we did with Tricia Thompson was, to me, one that we discussed for years. Because when we think historically about gluten-free food, oats have been problematic for years and years. And as we started advocating using more grains, based on studies that indicated the gluten-free diet was low in iron and B vitamins, of course the grains you'd look to are those ancient grains, quinoa and all that. But to me, in my head, if oats were potentially contaminated, is there no reason that all these other grains might potentially be contaminated? So when we did the study it was 32 samples. And of those, you know, close to one-third of them were contaminated. What that indicates, though, is just that there isn't the awareness in those other grains and in food production, that we really need to be careful about all ingredients coming into the gluten-free food. Interestingly, in Europe, in most of the gluten-free production facilities, every ingredient's tested before it's allowed into the production facility, so that you minimize that risk of cross-contamination. So the Europeans were well ahead of us in that case. But this was an important study because it brought to light that potential goes far beyond just oats. And we're now-- Tricia's continued to look at spices and other things that-- again, that potential risk may be there. We don't know for sure, but we have to research it and really see if it is.

But the production is probably less of a concern to the normal consumer than the consumer that buys that grain and takes it home and uses it themselves. Because if the grains are used in gluten-free production, that end product should be tested and therefore should be safe. But for the general consumer who's buying millet to increase, you know, the nutritional value of their diet or they're buying buckwheat or even soy flour, which is one of the most highly contaminated, to use in their home gluten-free products and things, that's where the real risk is involved. Because that consumer may get a batch, or may get flour that is contaminated. There is a solution. You need to look for products that are labeled gluten free, that say that they're tested or are certified. And then you know that those ingredients will be safe.

Tamar: What do you think is contributing to the prevalence of food allergies and sensitivities?

Anne: When we look at intolerances and allergies, there, I think, environment plays a role. And I think the role there can be environmental. When we look at what we're eating today, it's very different than what we ate 50 years ago. Fifty years ago, we ate less processed food. We ate seasonally, and we ate locally. So what happened is that you don't have foods that have as much of these common ingredients as you do now. You also had more variety, and you didn't eat as much of the same food year long. So now our food is almost a monoculture of certain core ingredients-- corn, wheat, soy-- so that we're exposed to higher amounts of them continually and from one source, so that where the body was not exposed to that high amount and that uniformity of ingredients, now we are. And I think that that may be a trigger that we really need to-- of course we need to research more and to really fine tune it.

Tamar: What's the difference between food allergies, intolerance and sensitivities, and what do you want people to know about the difference?

Anne: Because food intolerances are really based on the inability to break down that food. Lactose intolerance is probably the best example, where it's not that they are allergic to the protein in the food, but they just cannot break down the sugar, the carbohydrate in that. And that's what causes all those GI symptoms. So that when someone with an intolerance eats a food, it takes a little while for symptoms to occur because that food has to get to the gut where it can't be digested. And that's what causes resulting symptoms.

An allergy is actually an immune response to the protein in the food and it causes the body to create certain antibodies. They're different than the antibodies for Celiac disease. It's actually an IgE mediated response. And that's important because that response is sudden, severe but not long lasting, nor damaging long term. And that's an important thing. Whereas these people with allergies, it can be life threatening. Okay. And sudden. And people need to really respect that.

Celiac disease is different. It's an autoimmune response. So, again, it's that reaction to the protein in particular, but it's a different antibody pathway. It's an IgA mediated pathway. And what's important there is that it's not just a reaction to the food, but it causes this cascade of autoimmune responses that actually does cause damage long term. So while the symptoms may not happen as rapidly, the long-term effect can be devastating. And so it's really important that the body reacts differently. It's important for people to know how to respond in each case.

Tamar: Some people have both allergic reactions and intolerance to the exact same food.

Anne: Absolutely, just because you have one, doesn't mean you can't have another. What's important to realize in each of these different pathways, whether it's an allergy, an intolerance or Celiac disease, which is autoimmune, is that having one does not exclude you from having any of the others. So just because you have Celiac disease doesn't mean that you don't have, or couldn't have, a food intolerance. And potentially, as you said, it could be to the same ingredient, too, where you could be not only allergic to wheat, but gluten sensitive too. Most common is, what we find, is when the gut's affected in Celiac disease, that intestine is so damaged that it can cause reactions or inability to digest multiple other foods, and that's important that one doesn't exclude the other at all.

Tamar: Do you know anything about how they made decisions on what food allergies to list on packaging?

Anne: That was actually based from the FDA years and years ago. And they looked at the most common allergens at the time that were, again, through that evidence analysis process, the FDA uses the same process-- everyone does-- for research, and it was based on the prevalence and the severity of reactions. At that time, corn allergies and some of these others were not as common. And I think that, the good thing is, the FDA does review things and will, hopefully with enough consumer voices being heard, will look again at that, include more of those.

A great example of that, is that it was only a few years ago they added wheat to the common list of allergens, which wasn't there initially. There were only eight and then wheat was included. In the years since then, they actually then added gluten as a separate labeling altogether. So when you look at the allergen labeling, it was done years ago. 2004, they added wheat which was a new thing. And now they've moved forward with gluten-free labeling. So the more people that make their concerns known, it's always helpful. And that's not to say that there's nine on the label now, there might be 12 later.

Tamar: So gluten is still not listed under the list of allergens. It's an entirely separate thing.

Anne: It's an entirely separate labeling law.

Tamar: Why did they not just include it in the list of allergens?

Anne: Because again, it goes back to that differentiation between wheat as an allergy and gluten intolerance and Celiac disease being an autoimmune disease. So it's based on that. These are common allergens versus an autoimmune response to a food.

It causes a lot of confusion and concern. Because people may or may not be allergic to wheat, and yet they have to be gluten free. It makes it confusing for sure.

Tamar: What do you think of the current trend in people who are avoiding gluten even though they're not intolerant?

Anne: That always comes up and I honestly think, if you don't need to be gluten free, there's really no reason to do it. We did a study looking at the nutritional analysis of the gluten-free diet and unless you're careful and plan your meal well, it is nutritionally deficient in B vitamins, iron, calcium.

The joint study we did when we looked at people's intake, most people on a gluten-free diet do not meet the RDAs. There's been subsequent studies done both in the States and in Europe that looked at individuals on a gluten-free diet over time. And what we found, we found evidence in nutritional deficiencies. We found an increase weight gain of close to 20 pounds. We found all kinds of problems with people on a gluten-free diet. Now, when we looked at what people ate, unfortunately, going gluten free doesn't always mean eating healthy and well.

A standard gluten-free diet in the U.S. includes gluten-free donuts, gluten-free breads, gluten-free baked products, white rice, more white rice, more white rice, white rice-based products. Not things that are really the core of a gluten-free diet. When you look at the core of a gluten-free diet, it's a simple, wonderfully balanced diet. It's fruits and vegetables.

[39]

It's dairy products. It's meats. It's grains. Where the problem with the gluten-free diet comes in, from a nutritional aspect, and why we caution people against it, is that many people who start, who are diagnosed with a gluten intolerance or a gluten -related disorder, the things they tend to reach for are the things that are now on the forbidden list.

So we see an increased intake of cookies and baked items. And, as I'm sure you've met many people, they open a package of a gluten-free product, and not all of them are great and so they'll eat a cookie and say, "Well that wasn't that good." And then they'll eat another one hoping it'll get better, and then they'll finish the whole package and still not be satisfied. So that, obviously will lead to that weight gain. That's not a healthy diet.

We really are working very hard to get people to follow a healthy gluten-free diet doing things that are naturally gluten free-- using, you know, the gluten-free manufactured products in a reasonable amount and way, but also to include these grains that we talked about before, making sure that they are gluten free. But those are a wealth of nutrition that need to be in our diet.

So for someone who doesn't need to be gluten free, they don't need to get into this mess. They really have a great variety of food, and wheat based products actually offer a certain palatability, certain taste and texture in addition to the nutrition that they offer. So why would you give that up? If you're concerned about the amount of carbohydrates, choose different ones. Choose a variety. You don't need to be gluten free in order to have a healthy diet. And those that are gluten free, we need to do this much better.

Tamar: How do food allergies effect people physically, cognitively, emotionally? What's the most common reactions you see?

Anne: With food allergies and intolerances, it does effect a person on multiple levels. Physically, the inability to digest food will have an impact. But that physical response is going to affect them emotionally and therefore psychologically. When you are limited in what you can eat, it limits the rest of your life. When you think about when we enjoy food, what food is-- that common ground of getting together, of joining and sharing and socializing-- now that we've put a restraint on that, we've put a restraint on your life and your quality of life. And what we've found in the studies I've done on quality of life issues in the Celiac disease population, is that there is a diminished quality of life for many of these people. And it goes across age and gender. So it doesn't matter whether you're old or young there, you know, following a restricting diet limits your ability to enjoy that normal life. And I think that over time, although people tend to navigate and find out ways to kind of meet both needs physically as well as emotionally, it's still like that little chink every time you go out that, "Oh, I have to rethink this," or, "I have to really grill the waiter on how to do this."

And that will affect people psychologically long term. I think the one benefit of all the increased awareness of gluten free and the fad aspect of it is that people are more aware. The concern however is that it's perceived as a fad and not as a medical necessity. And that actually worries me that that may cause more damage, where it's, you're dismissed, as opposed to being recognized as someone who really needs to follow a diet for a medical reason.

I just finished a study in looking at quality of life-- scores of people who participate in different types of social support networks. And what we found is that those that participate in just online social support, whether it be a blog site, or chat rooms, or Facebook or things, actually had a lower quality of life score than those who participated in face-to-face support group meetings. And I think it goes back to having that feeling of support, of being surrounded by people that understand what you're doing. And I think that, you know, we need to look at it more deeply and do more research into some more of the nuances. Is it that real face-to-face support group meeting that's holding you up, or knowing that you have other people out there? So we'll follow up with that. But I think it's an interesting aspect that we now realize the importance of that contact or that acceptance in this whole area of food allergies and intolerances.

Aristo Vojdani, PhD, MSc, CLS. Interviewed 5/13/14

Tamar: Just talk for a second. Introduce yourself.

Aristo: I finished my Ph.D. in microbiology and immunology, then did post actual studies in the field of first comparative immunology, then tumor immunology. And so at certain level I got out of academia and decided to go into private industry.

Tamar: You don't use the terminology sensitivities or intolerance at all?

Aristo: I'm not. In fact, I'm talking about food immune reactivities. If it's not IgE mediated. Food immune reactivities. And/or immunities.

Tamar: What are the most common foods people react to?

Aristo: In relation to IgE mediated we know that nuts, seafood, corn, soy, milk, wheat, there are about eight major, major allergies. In the case of food immune reactivities, number 1 is wheat, number 2 is milk. And that will follow with corn and rice, whatever we consume more.

Tamar: Do you think that food allergies and sensitivities are more prevalent now or do you think that we're just more able to diagnose it now?

Aristo: I have no doubts they're more prevalent now. Because that actually, indirectly, saying that well, the pediatricians, were incapable 10 years ago, today they are capable and therefore can diagnose more

[43]

allergy or ADD or ADHD. I disagree with that. So yes, there is-- more ADD, more ADHD, more autism and more food allergy and sensitivities.

Tamar: Do you think that food allergies are going to reach epidemic proportions? And if so, what can we do before that happens, or do you think we're already there?

Aristo: We are already there. (shows magazine to me, *Trends In Immunology*) So the word epidemic is already in there. And they're talking about IgE mediated food allergy, which right now is about 7% of the population. But I believe it's much more than that. Much more than that. Maybe 20%.

Tamar: Is it just as bad in, do you know, in Europe or in other countries as it is in the U.S.?

Aristo: In the U.S. is the worst. Because in Europe, they already have many laws which take out many, many chemicals including some of the food colorings I was talking about. Bisphenol A, some of the cosmetics, they're not using. And so they are doing a better job there removing these chemicals and some of the pesticides. And so therefore yes, we are using more chemicals; and we have more allergies, sensitivities, and auto immunities.

Tamar: And what do you think is a major contributor to this?

Aristo: In general, we can say corn, and GMO and soy contribute to some degree. But in my opinion, because of my background, I believe the chemical triggers are playing much more of a role in development of allergies and auto immunities. Because, when you understand the mechanism of action, that all these chemicals, that after entering into our body, with the protein that we consume, those chemicals combine to the proteins and induce immune reactivity.

And so all the pesticides and chemicals which are in the food, get into the milk. And from the milk, obviously the chemicals combine to the protein of the milk; and now we are reacting to the combination of the pesticides plus the milk proteins such as alpha casein and beta casein.

Wheat, the same thing. And so I believe, one of the studies I did, published in a journal called *Nutrients*, I measured IgG, IgM, IgA, antibody non-IgE mediated immune reactivities. In 1,000 "healthy subjects," so called. 25% of them had very high levels of antibodies against milk and against wheat and its different components.

Why this is so important? Because the same antibodies are made against wheat proteins, cross-react with the cerebellum. And therefore "gluten ataxia"-- antibodies made against certain components of casein-- cross-react with GAD 65 eyelet cells and therefore type 1 diabetes and other neurologic disorders.

Tamar: What do you think of the current trend of people avoiding gluten, like it's a diet? People who aren't sensitive or haven't been tested at all.

Aristo: Well, I don't see any reason to be gluten free if you have no problem with it. But if you have a GI

[45]

problem or you have any immune disorders-- example, you know-- neurologic disorder, arthritis-- then I highly recommend. There are so many autoimmunities associated with gluten. If there's a history of immune disorders and auto immunities in the family, I highly recommend those individuals to be on gluten-free and dairy-free diet-- even currently do not have symptomatology. I'm not saying every human being on earth to be on gluten-free and dairy-free diet.

Tamar: They add food coloring to meat?

Aristo: Yes. Yes.

Tamar: That seems ridiculous. I'm just surprised by that. Nobody's said that before. So, it's interesting.

Aristo: Well, you know what is tandoori chicken? In India, what's tandoori chicken? Did you think it's saffron? Or paprika? No. Go online and check. It is food coloring. It's food coloring #5.

Dr. Vodjani is the founder of http://www.immunoscienceslab.com/ in Beverly Hills, CA.

ISL's founder is a professor of neuroimmunology at the Carrick Institute for Graduate Studies, a faculty member in the Dept. of Preventive Medicine at Loma Linda University, and a past associate professor at the Charles Drew/UCLA School of Medicine and Science. He obtained his M.Sc. and Ph.D. in the fields of microbiology and clinical immunology with postdoctoral studies in tumor immunology at UCLA. His on-going research, spanning a 45-year career, focuses on the role of environmental triggers in complex diseases. Professor Vojdani's research and focus on predictive antibodies has resulted in the development of numerous antibody arrays for the detection of many autoimmune disorders. Of particular note are the arrays for

[46]

autoimmune diseases that originate from the gut and manifest as attacks on the body's own tissues or organs, including the brain. An owner of 15 US patents for laboratory assessments, Professor Vojdani has published more than 140 articles in scientific journals. He is the CEO and Technical Director of Immunosciences Lab., Inc. in Los Angeles, CA, and sits on the editorial board of five scientific journals. In 2006, he was given the prestigious *Herbert J. Rinkel Award* by the American Academy of Environmental Medicine (AAEM) for excellence in teaching the techniques of environmental medicine. On November 7, 2009, he was given the *Linus Pauling, PhD Award* by the American College for Advancement in Medicine. And in October of 2012 he was given the ***F. R. Carrick Research Institute's extremely distinguished Lifetime Achievement Award***. (immunoscienceslab.com)

Doctor Alessio Fasano   Interviewed 8/1/14

Tamar: Give me your name. And, just talk about yourself for a minute. Just tell me where you're from, where we are right now?

Alessio: Alessio Fasano. I'm from Salerno, Italy. We're in Charlestown, Massachusetts at the Navy Yard that is the scientific hub of the Massachusetts General Hospital. And specifically, we're at the Center for Celiac Research and Mucosal Immunology and Biology Research Center at the Navy Yard.

Tamar: What made you originally turn your focus to food allergies and gluten?

Alessio: I'm a pediatric gastroenterologist by training. And my original interest was in diarrheal diseases. And actually, mainly acute diarrheal disease. The one due to infections. And because of my interest with gut physiology, I was very much focused how intestines react to an attack by bacteria. And over time my interest broadened to other conditions that lead to GI problems, particularly now gliadin. There's real diseases due to infections, much more rare than GI problems related to food intolerances in general.

And that was the reason why, eventually, slowly but surely this shift toward that direction. And then, you know, this went all in full circle. Because, you know, nutrition has been a great deal of interest in the past 10 years because the composition, the bacteria living in our guts, what we call the microbiome, is highly influenced by nutrition. And now we know that this bacteria can do so many good things to us, but also so many bad things to us. And that's the reason why the two go hand in hand.

Tamar: How important do you think labeling is? Because Europe seems to be ahead of us in terms of genetic modification labeling. Do you think that's helped their situation?

Alessio: Well, you know, definitely. Let's talk about GMOs first. They are not allowed in Europe, so they don't deal with the problem. Here, on the other hand, it's a little more relaxed law about this. Nevertheless, despite this discrepancy, the amount, the entity of the problem is pretty much the same. So, for me, this means, the genetically modified food stuff cannot be explaining this epidemics of problems we're witnessing here. There must be much more than that. Not disputing it could be a component but not the driving force of these huge problems that we see increasing over time. The labeling issue's extremely important when you have a specific sensitivity or intolerance for food stuff that is used, let's say, in food industry.

Gluten's the classical example. If it's used as filler or additive and you don't label the-- I don't know-- chicken or whatever that naturally should be gluten free, you don't know that you're exposed to gluten. So that's where I see the importance of the labeling.

Tamar: Well, if you don't think GMOs are really responsible at all, what do you think is responsible for this? Do you call it an epidemic or--?

Alessio: Oh, I really do believe there's an epidemic. Definitely for many food intolerances. And, let's call them food reactions. Because, when you have, intolerance, sensitivities and other forms of gluten reactions we're going to specifically discuss about mechanisms that are very, very different with different consequences. I think that again, when you have clinical outcomes, there are two possible explanations. Because the two key players are genes, i.e. your genetic predisposition to react to anything-- in this case, food stuff that goes the wrong direction. Or the environment. Something in the environment that is changing the outcome. The epidemic's-- because it's such, I think, we should talk. It occurred in such a short period of time that it is hard to believe that it's due to genetic modification of the human genome. That would take much longer. So gotta be the environment.

So we're changing the environment dramatically and fast enough that we cannot adapt. What in the environment? Well, we can discuss until tomorrow. You know, for sure the way that we eat. Only two generations ago, I want to say three generations ago, the refrigerator did not exist. So you have to eat stuff that's particularly perishable, that's produced locally and consumed within a certain period of time. Now we can eat stuff that has been harvested, you know, two years before. What that implies? What it's going to do to us? We are seasonally exposed to food stuff. Now there's no seasonality anymore. You can eat stuff all year round. Does this make a difference? We used to eat only stuff produced locally and existed locally. Now we can eat stuff produced in another corner of the globe. What that means? You know the bacteria comes on the surface of the stuff. Can they change the way they're risking outcome? This, just to name a few things related to nutrition.

But also they use and abuse antibiotics. The fact that we travel in real time from one part to another of the globe.

Tamar: So what do you think about the trend in so many people eating gluten free when they don't necessarily have a reason to, or they just think it's a fad diet or--?

Alessio: Brushing this off as a fad diet is a sin considering that the gluten-free diet for example is the cornerstone for the treatment for Celiac disease. It's like insulin for diabetics. You can't brush this off as a fad. I mean same for people, they suffer other gluten disorders like gluten sensitivity or wheat allergy. If they don't embrace a gluten-free diet they will be seriously sick. So if you don't embrace the gluten-free diet, again, you will be in jeopardy for great consequences. If you don't embrace the *South Beach Diet*, that's not the case. So you can't really make that kind of comparison.

Now, what is the element of truth-- that you feel better going gluten free or you lose weight going gluten free? There is no element of truth. Of course if you decide to go natural gluten free, so choose only a product that is naturally gluten free, now you're forced to eat healthy, to buy stuff that you need to cook yourself, because otherwise you don't know what is in there. And therefore choose whatever you put in your mouth and take the time to cook it. If you do that, of course you'll be healthy. The reason why, particularly

[51]

in the Western Hemisphere, we're paying the price, qualitative and quantitative price, of the consequence of an unhealthy diet is because we're in the fast lane of lifestyle. You ask my daughter recipes to cook, she will tell you the time that something goes in the microwave. That's for her, that's the cooking concept.

And because, if you have half an hour for lunch and you come home at 8:00 and you need to put everything on the table by 8:05, that's your option. But if you have to go gluten free, that option goes away. Or even worse, you stop by a fast food and you eat a sandwich there. You can't do that. So if that's what it's forcing you to do, eat gluten free, you will be healthier. But not because gluten free is healthier. Because you can have a healthy diet. You will eventually lose weight because you can't over feed yourself unless you purposely decide on huge portions of food stuff. Because, again, it's the intensity of the little sandwich that by itself seems to be not much, but you know there are sandwiches that can go all the way to 1,000 calories. If you cook it yourself to eat 1,000 calories, you will have three courses of stuff-- if you start with the salad, and then the rice and then some fish and meat. That's what it takes to get to that level. Now your belly's filled. Or, an unlimited amount of fruits and vegetables almost will bring you not even close to 1,000 calories.

And while gluten indeed, nutritionally, is useless, the consequence of going gluten free, if you don't do this right, depriving yourself for minerals, vitamins, fibers, can be, you know, detrimental. So you trying to fix something naturally, you end up to make stuff worse.

So I personally would never recommend to go gluten free unless 1) there is a rationale and 2) that you do so under the supervision of a dietician.

Tamar: Do you want to talk for a minute about the difference between Celiac disease and wheat allergy, sensitivities, intolerance?

Alessio: Roughly 1% of the general population is affected by the autoimmune response to gluten. Wheat allergy, on the other hand, is a food allergy, like allergies to peanuts or strawberries and so on and so forth. Same mechanism. The same steps at the beginning-- you eat gluten, gluten comes through the guts partially undigested as seen by the immune system, but now, rather than to activate the cascade of events that leads to autoimmunity.

Some of the symptoms can be overlapping with Celiac disease. Some are very, very different in that you know, you can go all the way to anaphylactic.

Then there's this third form of reaction that we call gluten sensitivity or non-Celiac gluten sensitivity in which there is still an immune response. It's not allergic. It's not autoimmune. So it's a different kind of response with a very similar clinical outcome. So they're all indistinguishable clinically.

Tamar: So then, do you find one of the reasons that this is happening to us so much is because gluten and corn and dairy and soy are in absolutely every single thing that we eat in trace amounts? Because, at one point you say in the book that our reaction to it is the same premise as vaccines. And, which is something I've been trying to tell people. It's in every single thing that we eat in trace amounts, so of course we're starting to build resistance to it.

Alessio: Definitely, the fact that we are exposed on a routine, daily basis to these food stuff can be one of the components why we have this clinical outcome. Is that the only component? I don't think so.

So, again, I'm not disputing the possibility that this increases level of exposure because everywhere can be part of it. But it cannot just be, just the end of the story. Because again, if you have the system that works fine, no matter how frequently you eat stuff, you should be just fine.

I mean, the typical example: In the Chinese civilization soy use is-- it's routine. On a daily basis they are exposed to soy. Particularly, until the recent past, that was part of their diet. They rarely got the problem. We, on the other hand, in the Western Hemisphere, we are much more susceptible to a reaction to soy. So you wonder, does the soy create the problem, is it something else that, under specific circumstances makes soy to shift from a friend, something that's good for us, to a foe, that is harming us? So. That's what I think makes more sense to me.

Tamar: You say in your book that gluten is not digestible by anyone. So, why are they putting it in everything?

Alessio: Well, because it's very palatable. It's very nice. The reason why we cannot digest probably gluten because we didn't evolve with that. For 2.5 million years We've been as a species gluten free for most of this time. So, the other thing is, that again, gluten is perceived when undigested, as an enemy by our immune system like we perceive bacteria. You deploy the same weaponry, at least we've seen so far, that you typically deploy when under attack from a microorganism that's like a bacteria.

Yet, very rarely we develop infections because there are very few times we lose the battle. The same as gluten. We eat gluten all the time. And very few people lose the battle. But the vast majority can eat that without consequences.

So, should we go all gluten free? I would say, if you go to that extreme, then we should all stop using cars because they pollute. Or, stop using cell phones because they can give you brain cancer. Or we can actually say, "You know what? Granted there are these risks. Why we don't make a better use and more logical use of this stuff?" So, we use the right gas in our car and we use the car only when we need it. Otherwise we use public transportation. We use the cell phone for communication not for chatting. We can do something else rather than stay three hours on the cell phone. By the same token say, rather than inundate us, all this stuff like gluten, can we eat that in a much more logical, moderated, balanced diet so that we minimize the risk? That's what in my humble opinion would be the logical approach.

World-renowned pediatric gastroenterologist, research scientist and entrepreneur Dr. Alessio Fasano is chief of Pediatric Gastroenterology and Nutrition at Mass General Hospital for Children (MGHfC). Dr. Fasano directs the Center for Celiac Research, specializing in the treatment of patients of all ages with gluten-related disorders, including

Celiac disease, wheat allergy and gluten sensitivity. He treats patients with acute and chronic diarrheal diseases, and treats infants and children who have difficult-to-treat gastrointestinal problems.

Dr. Fasano also directs the Mucosal Immunology and Biology Research Center and is associate chief for Basic, Clinical and Translational Research. Under his leadership, investigators are studying the molecular mechanisms of autoimmune disorders including Celiac disease, and other-gluten-related disorders. He has been named visiting professor of pediatrics at Harvard Medical School. He authored the groundbreaking study in 2003 that established the rate of Celiac disease at one in 133 Americans. Widely sought after by national and international media, Dr. Fasano has been featured in hundreds of interviews including outlets such as *The New York Times, The Wall Street Journal; National Public Radio; CNN; Bloomberg News*, and others. (http://massgeneral.org)

Author of *Gluten Freedom.*

Tom O'Bryan   Interviewed 5/3/14

Tamar: Tell me your name and where you're from.

Tom: Tom O'Bryan. Encinitas, California.

Tamar: And what's your background?

Tom: I'm on the teaching faculty at the Institute for Functional Medicine and a double board certified nutritionist. I was licensed as a chiropractic physician 30 years ago. I'm a certified functional medicine practitioner from the Institute of Functional Medicine, which is great. I'm also on the teaching faculty for the Institute of Functional Medicine. And in that role I teach about intestinal permeability, the leaky gut.

Tamar: What do you say to people that still think that Celiac disease or gluten sensitivity does not exist?

Tom: If anyone were to say Celiac disease does not exist I would be a little surprised. But then I would say, "Well, if you go to PubMed, which stands for Public Medical Information, pubmed.gov, it's the national library of medicine, and type into the search engine, 'Celiac disease,' you will have over 19,000 articles that pop up immediately." So, there are at least 19,000 research teams that have spent months of their lives reviewing some topic related to a subject that that person is saying doesn't exist. I would say that's not likely accurate.

Tamar: What is the difference between a food allergy and intolerance and a sensitivity?

Tom: Before 2011 there was no consensus in the world of Celiac research on a difference between allergies, intolerances, sensitivities and disease. There was no consensus, no agreement. In 2011 in Oslo, the International Celiac Symposium came up with an agreed upon series of terms and definitions. And they published that agreement in the *Journal of Gut* in 2012. And it's the nomenclature to use with gluten-related disorders. And they asked, "Could we all please use the same language? Could we all - all scientists, all researchers, all clinicians, all patients. Could we all be on the same page, please?"

And that is, that at the top of the umbrella, in the overview, the term is a "gluten-related disorder." Below that, if they have the genes and they have villous atrophy, it's "Celiac disease." And about 1% of the population has that. Depends on what group you're studying. If you're looking at first-degree relatives of Celiacs, it's as many as one out of five will have Celiac disease. But in general, it's one out of 100.

They've asked that we stop using the term "gluten intolerance" because it's very confusing to people. 'Cause people have heard of lactose intolerance and they know that if you have lactose intolerance that if you take lactase enzymes, you then can eat lactose without getting the bloating and the gas. So the term "gluten intolerance" suggests that people can take the enzymes that are out on the market and then go out and eat gluten. And they can't. And they will continue to have the same devastating diseases if they have that approach.

So, all of our experts agreed, "Please, can we stop using the world "gluten intolerance"? So there's Celiac disease, there's an allergy, which is an IgE reaction, then there's non-Celiac gluten sensitivity. Non-Celiac gluten sensitivity is-- they don't have Celiac disease, the endoscopy is negative, they don't have elevated transglutaminase antibodies, the biomarker in the blood for Celiac disease, but, they seem to get better if they go off gluten.

So, they-- that category of people have been referred to as non-Celiac gluten-sensitive people. The next category is wheat amylase trypsin inhibitors in wheat. That's where the book "Wheat Belly" comes into play that Dr. William Davis is addressing in his book very well. Well done. And he talks about the glycemic index of wheat - that it's higher than most fruit and that two slices of bread, you're body thinks it's eating a Snickers bar. That's how much insulin it produces. Two slices of whole wheat bread. So, that's why many people lose weight when they go on a gluten-free diet, is because they're stabilizing, they begin stabilizing their insulin levels and their blood sugar levels.

The next term is "FODMAP." The next category under gluten-related disorders is FODMAPs. And those are people who go gluten free, they feel a little bit better, but they don't feel great yet. And when they go off all grains they feel much, much better. So they have a problem with carbohydrates that are in wheat and other grains also. So they're much better off being grain free.

So, gluten-related disorder, Celiac disease, non-Celiac gluten sensitivity are the two main categories underneath that. And please stop using the word "intolerance." For all of us, stop using that word.

Tamar: What are some things that would surprise us?

Tom: Probably the most common link, with reproductive disorders, is a sensitivity-- food sensitivities. Not necessarily allergies, but food sensitivity of one type or another. And the most common food sensitivity was gluten and then dairy. Across the board. Almost every -- not quite everyone, but almost everyone-- which shows sensitivity. So, take those out, their body starts functioning better.

Tamar: How much of an increase in corn sensitivity are you seeing?

Tom: There's a couple of answers to that question. In the world of Celiac disease, what the studies suggest is that up to 50% of Celiacs also have a cross-sensitivity to corn. So that's a pretty high number. The other side of the answer to that question is the GMO part, which, almost all corn nowadays is GMO unless it's-- the manufacturers are very proud to say-- when it's not, 'cause it's more expensive to get it, right?

And, the studies have come out now that show that GMO will cause intestinal permeability, which is the gateway into the development of autoimmune disease. So any GMO foods have the potential of doing that.

Tamar: Is Celiac more prevalent now?

Tom: Currently today Celiac is four times higher than the numbers that had it back in the 1950s. So it's not the testing. There's almost a projected 400% earlier mortality now compared to the guys in the 1950s. So more people are getting sick and they're dying faster than we did 50 years ago-- 50 or 60 years ago. And the question is, "Why?"

What's happening now is that our immune system is activated so much earlier in life, there's so many more thousands of antigens, or things that offend the body and the immune system reacts to, there are thousands of antigens we're exposed to now every day, we weren't exposed to 60 years ago, 70 years ago. So our immune system is working overtime to try to protect us. Doing everything it can. So it's hypervigilant, it's on edge all the time now. And what happens at some point-- and this is why people who have a family member with Celiac and they get an endoscopy and they don't have Celiac at 22 years old-- this is why they develop Celiac at 40-- or 45. And they get an endoscopy and now they've got Celiac. It's, well, they always had the risk, but now they've got the villous atrophy. And it's because they've crossed the threshold. And it's a loss of oral tolerance. We no longer can tolerate this antigen anymore. And the body cannot fight it. It just can't deal with it anymore. And that's because of the GMO foods, the antibiotics we're exposed to, the chemicals, the pesticides, the vaccinations, the bad air, the toxic chemicals in the carpets that we have in our home-- it goes on-- the heavy metals in the water, in the fish, etcetera.

Tamar: So, do you think it's going to reach epidemic proportions?

Tom: Oh my goodness. It's already epidemic proportions. If you look at non-Celiac gluten sensitivity, do the right test, clinically what you find is somewhere between 40 to 60% of the people that come into your practice will come back positive on sensitivity to gluten. If you do the right test. In the general public, it's around 20 to 30%. But the ones that come to see you are the ones that are sick. So in that population it's 40 to 60%. They're positive.

Tamar: Yet there are so many people that are intolerant or sensitive and have absolutely no idea because they think whatever they are like, is what's normal.

Tom: Exactly. I just had a conversation with a gal after my presentation today. She says, "You know, I mean, why is gluten a problem? I mean, I have the gene, but I don't have a problem with gluten. I know I don't." I said, "Well, you're Hashimoto's though, aren't you?" And she, "How did you know?" And I said, "Well, I can see it. You know, it's obvious. But that may be how it's manifesting for you. It's not manifesting in the gut with what we think are the classic symptoms."

For every one person that's got GI symptoms, there are eight that don't. They have symptoms somewhere else in their body-- their thyroid, their brain, their knees. Startling how many people have a reaction that affects their brain. Startling. It's the most common system I have found clinically that's affected by a sensitivity to gluten.

Tamar: What would surprise us to learn?

Tom: Well, first about the term "allergy." You can only use the term allergy if you have an IgE reaction. That's the pin pricks. You also can do IgE in the blood but the more common way is the pin prick. Now that's the first test for allergies that ever was designed, back in the 1950s. And there was a subspecialty in medicine that really wrapped their heads around that one and they were called "allergists." And so they came up with definitions, really delineated well what the mechanism is, how it occurs-- when you eat a food, it causes this histamine reaction in your body, that's an allergy. So we can't call any other type of immune response an allergy. So we have to stop referring to food allergies, unless we're talking about an IgE reaction.

And it's confusing when you're trying to have a discussion differentiating different types of immune responses. We have an Army, Air Force, Marines, Coast Guard, Navy. IgG, IgA, IgE, IgM-- they're all different. They all have different purposes.

The next startling surprise that most people don't think about is that when you check for food sensitivities, some people will do an IgG test. And they'll do 90 foods and you'll get it for a few hundred dollars. It's a good price, and you look at 90 foods. If the food, IgG food allergy test comes back negative, it doesn't mean that that food's okay. It just means that the Army has not responded. What about the Navy? It may be an IgA reaction, or an IgE reaction.

We just published a paper on IgE reactions in Meniere's disease, to gluten. And we found that there were many people that did not have an IgE reaction-- they had Meniere's disease-- but they had an IgG or an IgA reaction. They didn't have an allergy, an IgE reaction, but they had a non-Celiac gluten sensitivity immune response.

So, when you do a test to look for food sensitivities, you can't do just one immunoglobulin, like IgG or IgE. If you do just IgG, if it's positive, it's positive. It's positive. But if it's negative, it may be that you have an Army reaction and you have to check IgA.

Tamar: A doctor in New York a few weeks ago was saying how you can have a food allergy and a sensitivity to the same exact food.

Tom: The Army and the Air Force are both out.

Tamar: Did you know that in New York State they just outlawed doing a full allergy workup? You can't do food testing, period, anymore-- in New York.

Tom: That's politics. New York's the only state in the union where you have to have the lab in the state to offer the test in the state. You can't be an outside lab. That's just all politics.

Tamar: Yeah. Do you know of any other states that that's happening?

Tom: No. That's just New York. And New Yorkers are letting it happen.

Tamar: New Yorkers don't even know that it's happening.

Tom: Well, someone needs to get mad enough and do a public education campaign then you go after the legislators. And you just make sure the legislators understand that you're not gonna vote for them if they do that again.

Dr. Tom O'Bryan is an internationally recognized speaker and workshop leader specializing in the complications of Non-Celiac Gluten Sensitivity and Celiac Disease as they occur inside and outside of the intestines. He is the founder of www.theDr.com. He recently hosted the paradigm-shifting The Gluten Summit – A Grain of Truth, bringing together 29 of the world's experts on Celiac Disease and Non-Celiac Gluten Sensitivity at www.theglutensummit.com. (thedr.com)

Alexander R. Shikhman, MD, PhD, CEO &
Founder IFSMED - Care For Arthritis &
Autoimmune Diseases   Interviewed 5/3/14

Tamar: So, the first question is: What made you turn your focus to food allergies and intolerance?

Alex: So, basically I've been practicing here in the States for over 17 years and I'm rheumatologist and I have a degree in immunology. I'm PhD in immunology. So I found that as a specialist in autoimmune diseases and rheumatic diseases it's difficult to complete the healing process without paying attention to the diet. And so around 10 to 12 years ago I start playing with various diets and I came across gluten-free diet and I noticed that it can make a huge difference in my patients' lives. And that's how the story started.

Tamar: Why do you think that food allergies are more prevalent now, or do you think they're more prevalent now?

Alex: You know, it's a tough question. So, first of all, we don't have clear statistics. So yes, we do think that they are more prevalent. And the question is, "Why?"

The first answer is because people pay more attention to what they eat. Right? So we're a little more cautious about what we eat. And we pay more attention between symptoms which we have and food which we eat, right? So it's - all the news. So I think that to some degree it's a matter of people being a bit more educated, right? So that's number one.

Number two, the food which we eat now probably different compared with the food which we ate 20, 30 years ago. And definitely it's different from the food which our parents and grandparents ate. Right? So, we're dealing with much more food additives right now, so that's number one. We're dealing with genetically modified foods, which is number two. And we're dealing with a whole range of antibiotics and hormones and other things which basically is used to raise cattle and, you know, whole poultry industry and things like that. So it's a tough question but probably it's an interplay.

Tamar: Do you think the more genetically modified food we have the more we're gonna see food allergies?

Alex: It's a good question. Probably. Again, I don't have a straight answer, but if I would guess so, probably yes, because genetically modified food is not the food which our ancestors ate and our body genetically cannot handle it appropriately.

So, typical example is the gluten. So genetically modified wheat has much, much high concentration gluten than the wild wheat, right? And probably it's one of the explanations why more and more people have gluten intolerance.

But again, you know, there's not very straight scientific studies; it's just my gut feeling.

Tamar: What do you find is the difference between food allergies, intolerance and sensitivities?

Alex: So, definitely there is a difference between food allergy and food intolerance. So, food allergy, it's an immediate reaction. You eat something and you feel the consequence of what you ate almost instantly. Forms of typical allergic reactions such as skin rash, hives, things like that. So, food intolerance, it's more a delayed type of response and you can feel the consequence somewhere from an hour or thirty minutes down to a couple of days. So it's a completely different response.

Food sensitivity in my mind is identical to food intolerance. Or maybe it's a hybrid between food intolerance and food allergy. So from my standpoint I don't use food sensitivity more because, again, it's not. It's not the exact term which I like because there's a huge response which is allergy, there's a delayed response which is intolerance, and sensitivity is something in between.

Tamar: How do you find that food allergies and intolerance affect people both physically, emotionally and cognitively? What are the most common signs that you see?

Alex: The most common problem which I see in my practice is fatigue. So most of the patients in my practice who have, for example, gluten intolerance or any type of other food intolerance, it is not true allergy but intolerance, they experience fatigue. And the fatigue starts somewhere between 15 to 20 minutes and it lasts up to several hours after consuming of inappropriate food. Right?

So, the other symptoms which we see-- joint pain, muscle pain, headaches-- so, which can last for a couple hours up to days.

Tamar: And brain fog?

Alex: Oh, brain fog and fatigue, they're kind of interconnected. Yes, absolutely.

Tamar: Interesting. So if somebody falls asleep right away?

Alex: It's a fatigue.

Tamar: Is that an intolerance or is that an allergy?

Alex: It's not an allergy. It's intolerance by my definition.

So while we're talking about allergy in my mind, my imagination, almost instantly creates an image that it's kind of hives. So it's more or less kind of skin reaction. It's swollen lips. So it's basically in scientific terms, IgE mediated process. Right? So you have much more kind of histamine type of reaction.

Tamar: But people can actually have the same-- they can have intolerances--

Alex: Yes. Yes absolutely. Yes.

Tamar: --and allergies to the same kind of foods. Do you have any food issues personally?

Alex: I decided to go gluten free because I have family-- my mother actually suffered from gluten intolerance for a long time and she passed away from complications from this condition. And I decided voluntarily to get rid of gluten over ten years ago. So

[69]

I've been gluten free for over ten years. And now, when I have some gluten, my typical manifestation, I need to take a nap. Because I don't have any other symptoms but I feel extremely fatigued.

Actually my wife bought me a barley-based broth a couple months ago so I had to call up my clinic because I had to take a nap. I couldn't function. (CHUCKLES) But again, the longer you stay off the gluten the more you feel the reaction. So I compare it when I talk to my patients compared to alcohol-- if you drink constantly, you're constant drunk. So you drink more or less, doesn't matter, you're drunk, right? Then you go sober, so, and then you stay sober for a while. And then you drink a little bit, and you feel huge effect of the alcohol. It's the same true for gluten and other things.

Tamar: Can you tell me more about prolamine intolerance?

Alex: Well, prolamines are proteins which are reached in proline. So these are proteins which our body cannot digest completely. And again, based in my estimation, 10 to 20% of people who have gluten intolerance, they have also intolerance to prolamines. And these are the people who have issues dealing with corn and oats and rice. And so these are people who have a very tough life because, again, there are not many products which they can consume.

Tamar: Is there anything that we would be surprised to learn? Anything that you really want to say to make sure the information is out there?

Alex: No, it's just basically the physicians need to be a bit more educated and they need to start introducing the whole idea that food affects your health in the routine medical practice. Because right now it's ridiculous that I have patients, when they go to physicians, this is kind of a forbidden question. Physicians don't want to talk about that. And they end up seeing chiropractors and people who are not qualified to do all these things, from my standpoint. So it's a pure medical issue-- and I don't know why-- it needs to be a kind of mainstream, one of the mainstream medical community. So, I don't understand why physicians are so resistant. So.

The only few physicians who I know who kind of share my philosophy, they have great results. And again, it's like treating patients with no medications, right? To some degree. Especially in the diet, you know, it helps with your illnesses. What else can you mention? That's the greatest satisfaction, right? So I don't understand it.

It's kind of conservatism of medical thinking. Probably, maybe it's a part of education. So I think that if we can approach medical schools, start talking to, you know, deans of medical schools about introducing a course of, let's say, medical nutrition, or nutrition and human disease, or something like that, because it starts from medical school.

Dr. Shikhman is board certified in internal medicine and rheumatology. He is a leading author of numerous scientific publications in peer review journals, including *Journal of Immunology*, *Arthritis and Rheumatism*, *Annals of Rheumatic Diseases*, *New England Journal of*

Medicine, Journal of Gluten Sensitivity and *Nature Biotechnology,* among others.

He is listed in *Who is Who in American Medicine and Healthcare* and *America's Top Physicians* by Consumer's Research Council of America. His other awards include a research grant from the Oklahoma Center for the Advancement of Science and Technology, an Oklahoma University award in clinical excellence, and a Skaggs scholarship in biomedical research.

Currently, Dr. Shikhman serves as a member of the editorial board of Future Rheumatology/International Journal of Clinical Rheumatology and is an advisory board member of *Simply Gluten Free* magazine.

Dr. Shikhman received his MD Cum Laude from the Russian State Medical University (formerly known as 2nd Moscow Medical Institute named after Pirogov) — a preeminent Russian medical center. After graduating from medical school, he spent five years in basic and clinical research in the area of autoimmune diseases driven by infectious agents and received his Ph.D. in Immunology from the Moscow Medical Academy (formerly known as 1st Moscow Medical Institute named after Sechenov).

In 1990 he immigrated to the United States and became a research professor at the Oklahoma University Health Sciences Center, Oklahoma City, where he conducted pioneering work on mechanisms of molecular mimicry between streptococcus group A and human skin proteins. He served his internship and residency in internal medicine at the Oklahoma University Health Sciences Center and completed his clinical fellowship in rheumatology at Scripps Clinic. Subsequently, he became a member of Scripps Clinic Division of Rheumatology and a faculty member in the Department of Arthritis Research at the Scripps Research Institute. His additional training included: study of medical acupuncture at UCLA, master classes in musculoskeletal ultrasound, auricolotherapy and auriculodiagnosis, and application of low-level lasers in therapy of arthritis and allied conditions.

Dr. Shikhman was among the first awardees of the National Institute of Complementary and Alternative Medicine to study the molecular mechanisms of glucosamine in arthritis. His research resulted in the discovery of glucose transporting mechanisms in human cartilage tissue and identification of several natural products with promising therapeutic benefits for patients with osteoarthritis.

As a symbiosis of his clinical and basic research activities, Dr. Shikhman developed a comprehensive approach to treat various arthritic conditions which combines state-of-the-art diagnostic and therapeutic modalities, dietary modifications, nutritional supplements and biomechanical adjustments. (ifsmed.com)

Tamar: Tell me your name and where you're from.

Stephen: I'm Doctor Stephen Wangen from Seattle, Washington, and I'm the medical director of the IBS Treatment Center. We're located in Los Angeles as well as Seattle. I wrote a book called *Healthier Without Wheat* that has been a very popular book on helping people understand the differences between Celiac disease and gluten sensitivity.

Tamar: So explain to me IBS.

Stephen: IBS stands for Irritable Bowel Syndrome and really what it is, is a label that just describes a multitude of digestive problems that essentially get no answer. So if you have diarrhea or you have constipation, or you have abdominal pain, or gas or bloating, in any combination-- some people have all of them, some people just have one-- if you have that, you're likely to get labeled with IBS assuming you don't have anything else. So typically everything else is ruled out, and that's what you're left with.

Tamar: So, what are some of the possible reactions to food that you see?

Stephen: There are many, many different reactions that you can have to a food. Those can vary from anything from headaches to joint pains, to digestive problems of all types, to chronic anemia, to osteoporosis. You name it. If there's a health problem, it probably can be tied in to a food reaction.

Tamar: What are the statistics of people that have IBS that don't know it?

Stephen: There are many, many people that suffer from IBS and don't realize it. We know that at least 15% of the population has IBS, but probably most people don't call it that.

Tamar: What are the number of people that have a food allergy or food intolerance and don't know it?

Stephen: The number of people that have a food allergy or food intolerance is probably staggering. We don't really have statistics on this, but in my estimation it's probably half the population.

Tamar: Why do doctors not automatically think of or test patients for food reactions?

Stephen: Doctors are not trained to think in terms of food reactions being the cause of their patients' symptoms. So that is why I think they really don't look for it in most patients and don't test for it.

Tamar: Why-- you say this in your book-- why is skin testing not helpful in detecting food reactions?

Stephen: Skin testing isn't helpful for discovering most food reactions, because it only applies to that really limited number of symptoms that most allergists think about, which is anaphylaxis, hives, eczema, asthma and allergic rhinitis. It's helpful in those areas, but it's not helpful when you're looking for any of the other kinds of reactions that you could have to food.

Tamar: You write about the limits of taking lactose enzymes for lactose reactions. Can you expand on that?

Stephen: In my experience, most people that react to dairy, do not have a lactose intolerance. And there's a real clear distinction in those areas. A lactose intolerance is an enzyme deficiency. A lactose intolerance can only cause some gas, bloating, and some digestive distress. You have to have a dairy allergy to cause anything else. Because you have to have an inflammatory reaction. And a lactose intolerance is not an inflammatory reaction. It's an enzyme deficiency. So if you're taking a (digestive enzyme) pill to digest your lactose, or you're drinking lactose-free milk, that won't help you if you have one of these broader inflammatory issues to dairy that cause things like congestion and headaches and all kinds of other problems, for example, like gluten can.

Tamar: How much do genetics play a part in the number of food intolerances?

Stephen: I think that genetics are a huge issue when it comes to food reactions and food intolerances. I see, in my patients, in family members, a lot of overlap and similarity in the kinds of food that they react to. So I think it's something that that genetic predisposition has carried on, has passed on. Just like it is in Celiac disease, it is for other food reactions as well. You tend to see a higher incidence in kids and other family members.

Tamar: Do you have any food allergies, sensitivities, intolerances?

Stephen: I am reactive, I am gluten intolerant and I also react to dairy, which, for some reason we call an allergy, but they're the same kind of thing. They're both immune reactions to the food.

And I don't eat gluten. I haven't for 19 years now. But I also remember as I was younger I would get acne. I would get-- I remember my hands would swell up for no reason. I just had a lot of brain fog, fatigue. I was supposedly very healthy because I was very athletic. But I now realize I wasn't as healthy as I should have been.

Dr. Stephen Wangen is the co-founder and Medical Director of the IBS Treatment Center. He is a licensed and board certified physician with a doctoral degree in naturopathic medicine and a bachelor's degree in biology, with honors. He is the award winning author of two books on solving digestive disorders, and a nationally recognized speaker. He has been seen and heard on ABC, NBC, and Fox as well as public radio and television. He was recently named one of Seattle's Top Doctors by Seattle Magazine.

His passion for being a doctor and solving digestive problems comes from a lifelong obsession with optimizing health. Having suffered from IBS as a young man, Dr. Wangen dedicated his life to solving this complex problem. He now hand picks and oversees other fine doctors at the IBS Treatment Center for the new specialty of IBS medicine. Since 2005 the IBS Treatment Center, with locations in both Seattle and Los Angeles, has successfully helped thousands of patients from around the country and the world end their digestive problems. (http://IBSTreatmentcenter.com)

He is also the writer of *Healthier Without Wheat* and *The Irritable Bowel Syndrome Treatment*.

Alicia: I'm Alicia Woodward. I'm editor and chief of Living Without's *Gluten Free & More* magazine.

Tamar: You recently changed the name of the magazine. So what made you suddenly decide to change it?

Alicia: We had always been focused a lot on disease. The original magazine, when it was first launched in 1998 by Peggy Wagner and I-- was the first editor-- our focus at that point was disease and going gluten free. So we didn't want to lose that focus, but we were trying to think of a way of saying disease, gluten-free lifestyle, food-friendly food, food-allergic living and say it in a positive way.

We had always tried to say that *Living Without* was living without gastrointestinal symptoms, living without deprivation, living without illness. But I think that overall, when anyone heard about the magazine for the first time, sometimes the reaction was, "Oh, your title's so negative." So we've been thinking actually, since the thing was launched in 1998, even the original creator was like, "Is there a better way to say this?" And so finally, we decided it was really time to launch this.

And so we stayed with our-- the whole *Gluten Free & More* is to encompass our original mission which is for the community, the gluten-sensitive community and also the food-allergic community. So we hope that the name just kind of describes exactly who we are in a very positive way. Because that's who we are. That's how we feel this community should be living.

Tamar: What are some of the critical things that you think need to happen?

Alicia: There's a lot of policy changes that need to be done. First of all, FDA's labeling that's coming, gluten-free labeling is great. It's coming into effect in August (2014). Those are the kinds of things like, we were on Capitol Hill lobbying for that and working on that. But so much more needs to be done in terms of epinephrine, having that readily available in the schools. The whole issue of school nurses in the schools-- a lot of these schools aren't covered and kids are dying because there's no trained medical staff at the schools.

The issue of food allergies and gluten-free food being expensive and treatment not being available for people who are lower income and don't have terrific resources-- it's a crying need. It's a crying need for these kids that are really sick, that these families where parents have to work two or three jobs or whatever. I mean, even the people with the best resources, whose kids come down with these allergies or sensitivities, they're totally thrown for a loop. I mean, even doctors with all of that background and stuff like, "Oh, my goodness," so how much more difficult for families or single moms or that kind of thing. And these kids aren't getting good care. So it's this kind of thing that, you know, we need to change. We need to make, you know, the country more aware of these pressing needs.

Tamar: What are your thoughts on corn sensitivity?

Alicia: Did you know that even 10 or 15 years ago corn wasn't considered a food that you could have an allergy to? When I first started this magazine and the person who was in charge of FAAN: Food Allergy and Anaphlaxis Network in Fairfax, Virginia-- her name was Ann Munoz-- I basically interviewed her and she said, "You know, there's really no evidence that there is a corn allergy." It's not that she was wrong; it's that the food supply has changed so much. And now corn is, although it's not in the big eight, you know, people are really reactive to it. And why is that?

I think we're changing the composition of some of our primary ingredients including corn. I think it's a multifactorial thing actually. First of all, the whole issue of genetic engineering where they're inserting bacteria or whatever in order to make these major food items withstand herbicide. The Roundup herbicide. Glyphosate.

It's changing. We don't know the ramifications of what's happening with these foods. It's basically corn, soy and sugar are the 3 big ones. Those ingredients are in almost everything we eat. Every processed food we eat. So the jury's out about that. We're kind of having this experimentation on our food supply. We don't know what the effects of that are.

And there's a strong lobby against even labeling of these ingredients and it's been rather alarming for me to watch that. Because to me it seems pretty ethical to label our products like what's in it, what's not in it.

The other issue is a lot of this-- the Roundup is being sprayed on all of these plants and that's, I think, how wheat is involved as well, 'cause it gets a lot of that massive spraying. I mean, I own a 250-acre farm, so we get a lot of the farm journals. And I mean, these farmers are complaining because we're developing these super weeds that can withstand these herbicides. And so, what do we do? We just spray more and more of it. And that's part of our food supply. Then we're all ingesting this stuff. In addition to that, I think we're changing the biome of what's going on in our bodies. And I think this has happened over multiple generations, where you have people who are using a lot of-- we've been using antibiotics, you know, without impunity. Mothers haven't been nursing and we're almost C section on-demand now.

And so we're losing that rich biome that, you know, we've had for thousands of years. And we've changed that so quickly and changed our food supply so quickly that I don't think we've evolved to be digesting a lot of the things that we're eating, and I think it's causing us a lot of trouble. I think it's very complicated. And there's a lot of different issues involved, and I think we're just now beginning to wake up to the implications of what's going on.

Tamar: And what do you think about people who adapt a gluten-free lifestyle that aren't at all intolerant?

Alicia: That is a huge trend. I find it fascinating. I find it so fascinating. In a million years I never would have predicted that that would be occurring and so quickly. When we first started this magazine, you had to spell

[81]

the word, "Celiac". You had to spell "gluten." You had to explain it to people. I mean, you couldn't find any food out there. The manufacturers of gluten-free food, you know, you could count them on one hand.

And now that everybody knows what gluten is. Even in rural areas, they've heard of it. So it's kind of exciting. In a way it's a wonderful thing because the market is booming, the products are just out there. You can go to your local grocery store. You know, you go to a restaurant and people are aware of it. And in public schools people are aware of it. And so I love that heightened awareness. When we first started the magazine, we were rolling the boulder uphill to try to get people aware to what disease was.

Now the downside to that is, that it's SO popular, that I think there's a lot of confusion about how strict do you have to be on this diet. And the spectrum of gluten sensitivity is really wide, and we haven't really figured that out yet. It's just kind of a new entity. And so we haven't even defined it yet in a way of biomarkers. So you can eat gluten and maybe feel foggy-brained. Or you can eat gluten and develop, you know, major intestinal damage.

And you're still all considered gluten free, or you can just go on the gluten-free diet because you think that might help you lose weight. And every one of those people is considered gluten free. And so the marketplace is serving every single one of those people. I think that will shake out. I think that the people who are doing it now because it's kind of a fad, I think that will calm down a little bit. We're kind of in a frenzy right now.

So I think generally it's a great thing, but it is adding to the confusion. And maybe it might even be adding to some of the safety issues. On the other hand, it's alerted the FDA to this kind of issue. And I think it's prompted even more studies into what's going on with reactivity to gluten. So I think overall it's a good thing.

It's an underrepresented population. And I think lately, for all the good joking about things on the late night shows, and the cartoons and stuff like that, it's funny, OK? It's funny. I laugh. But there's an undercurrent to that of dismissiveness that's dangerous. I have a great sense of humor. And I think we should all, you know, roll with this. But I don't want us ever to think this isn't god-awful serious for people who are sick. I mean, this is serious business. It's no joking matter. So, yeah, that's kind of where we stand with the magazine.

Tamar: I'm sure that you've learned already that every person who-- especially people who've been diagnosed with any sort of intolerance years ago-- everybody has done all this research on their own. So it's just a very well-informed community. And they're very supportive of each other. And, there's so much more information out there now than there used to be. But every person who this happens to, they suddenly realize that they have to change everything about their lifestyle.

Alicia: Okay. That's a good point. That can't be overstated. In other words, the reason we're such a tight community is because everybody's kind of thrown out there by themselves. There's so much naysaying, even by the medical-- especially by the medical community. And there's so much like, "This is in your head," or, "You're overreacting," or, "This is another hysterical woman with, you know, chronic fatigue syndrome, or some other kind of umbrella thing," that it's all histrionic.

And so when you get these people who are really sick, and they're doing their own research, and they're trying this and that, and they finally discover, and then they find somebody else, you have this instant intimacy with these people. And it's an amazing bond. But in my mind, that's a reflection on the fact that we still have a long way to go to inform the medical community so that we're not all out there doing our own research alone.

And there's a panic to that. OK? Especially if it's your child, and your child's not well, and you see your child going down the tube, and the doctors are saying, "Well, she'll grow out of it," or something. I mean that, that kind of panic and terror is unimaginable for that mother. And then it's like revamping everything you ever thought about in terms of food and diet and how you cook. I mean, it's completely overwhelming. So. Yeah. I mean, your heart breaks for this community.

On the other hand, you get goose bumps of excitement to see the courage and strength in the community, and to see these parents fighting for their kids, or someone who's been sick for years, like, "Gosh, darn it! No more." You know? So yeah, there's a lot of-- everyone has a story and they're all so inspiring. So you look at this community, it's like, these people are heroes. They're unsung quiet heroes. Shoot, we want to honor that. We need to honor that.

I think what's also exciting is this whole heritage wheat thing. Okay. So people are starting to go back to the original wheat that was used 100 or 200 years ago either from overseas Eastern European countries or from some of these seed banks where they've kept these older seeds. And it's now, there's now more and more-- these are not peer review studies in medical journals, but there's more and more anecdotal evidence now that people who have non-gluten sensitivity can eat wheat from this heirloom wheat, this old wheat. And that's pretty exciting too. If you hear these stories, and you have these people making these claims, and also these companies now that are-- so there's more companies now, more farmers growing these old seeds, more companies now baking bread with these old flours. So I think that's a neat trend that we're going to see and that's extremely exciting.

And I think the other thing that's interesting that I'm waiting to see happen is, it's not just food allergies that are being impacted by the way-- whatever it is in our environment. I tend to think it's the way we've altered our food, but maybe the way we've altered our biome and all of these things. But, you're seeing these epidemic-raising increases in autism, in Asperger's, in asthma, in autoimmune diseases, in ADHD. So there's a proliferation of these autoimmune kind of-- other kinds of behavioral disorders. So I'm very interested to see how a lot of the studies about gluten and food allergies will be impacting on these other populations as well. I think there's a definite link.

Gluten Free & More's editor, Alicia Woodward, LCSW, a licensed psychotherapist, blogs about upcoming articles and topics being prepared for the magazine--everything from gluten-free life stories to the medical research and breakthroughs on Celiac disease. Alicia also comments on letters and feedback received from readers on gluten-free living. (http://glutenfreeandmore.com)

Mary: My name is Mary Capone and I am the founder and manufacturer of Bella Gluten-Free products as well as cookbook author. I have two cookbooks actually-- one that I did with *Living Without*, the celebrity chef edition, and also my first cookbook was *Gluten-Free Italian Cookbook*, which is still going quite strong. And I had a cooking school.

Tamar: What made you start this school?

Mary: I had found out I was a Celiac and then I went right back into my kitchen and started recreating all my old family recipes which are primarily Italian. My last name is Capone. And I just started thinking, "I need to bring this information to people." And that was back in 2005 when I started the school. I really wanted to bring a gourmet feel to this diet. And when I found out, it was particularly gluten free at the beginning. But what I found out is that people had multiple allergies. They had dairy, they had corn, they had soy. So we basically did an allergen-free cooking school and fantastic food came out of that.

Tamar: Who was the first person to diagnose you?

Mary: I was diagnosed by a naturopath. And then I was diagnosed later by a gastroenterologist. But I took myself off of the gluten for about a year and a half before I was actually diagnosed with Celiac disease. I had, you know, several autoimmune diseases that cleared up beautifully when I went on this gluten-free diet.

Tamar: Nice. Are you allergic to anything else?

Mary: Yes. Corn. I'm not a big fan of corn. I think that the GMO has really ruined that product, or that crop-- because of the cross-pollination. So I don't put any corn in my manufactured ingredient, you know, packaging, my mixes. I don't put any soy in there either. So I think people are reacting to corn a lot more than they used to. And, you know, dairy, I'm lactase, lactose intolerant. And not casein. So what I found out when I was doing that cooking school was that people are allergic to usually more than one thing.

Tamar: Is there anything that you think would surprise us to learn? Is there anything you want to get out there?

Mary: I think, you know, people will try this diet and do it three-quarters of the way or 90% of the way, and what I've learned is that it's so important to do it 100%. Because your body will still react as if you took, from one crumb, the same reaction as a whole loaf of bread. So that army of antibodies will come in and flood your system and cause inflammation and a lot of damage to the tissue as the immune system is hunting down that gluten molecule and trying to kill it. It kills a lot of other things, or injures a lot of other things along the way. So I think that's really interesting. People always say, "Well, I'm almost all gluten free." Well no, you have to be 100%. And, that one crumb, one single crumb equals 20 parts per million. So it's really important to not use-- not cross-contaminating your environment-- so using a separate toaster if you're dealing with a kitchen where people are eating wheat and not.

Diagnosed with celiac disease, our founder, Mary Capone combines her gluten-free mastery with her love of the kitchen to create scrumptious gluten-free, allergen-free cuisine. Mary is a cookbook author, and nationally known instructor of gourmet gluten and allergen-free foods. As a celiac chef with celiac kids, Mary has designed mixes that not only have great taste and texture but include plenty of healthy ingredients as well. Her articles and recipes have appeared in *Living Without Magazine, The Herb Quarterly, Energy for Women, Eatingwell.com, Livingwithout.com, Delicious Living Magazine and Delight Gluten-Free*. Her book, *The Gluten-Free Italian Cookbook* includes over 141 delicious gluten-free classic Italian recipes with 135 allergen-friendly variations. (http://BellaGlutenFree.com)

Former Maine dairy farmer Peter Paton
Interviewed 4/6/14

Tamar: Peter, you were a dairy farmer growing up in Maine. But what were you telling me about corn?

Peter Paton: I'm becoming concerned about our beef supply. Because more and more of it is coming from large scale farms who have a feedlot approach to feeding their livestock. And they're just trying to get as much feed into the animals as they can, in order to get their body weight up. And so I have to wonder if it's the best possible food for humans, nutrition wise. And there's so much corn being fed, I'm concerned about the fact that our corn supply is becoming genetically modified. And if this is the primary source of feed for our beef cows, and what does that say about our supply of beef. It's almost like the beef industry is becoming nothing more than a vehicle to get the corn from the corn field to the consumer. Cause that's primarily what the beef cows eat. And our corn supply, especially for livestock feed, is certainly becoming genetically modified.

Tamar: What concerns you about that?

Peter: Because you see, the genetically modifying process is unnatural. We're breeding things that aren't normally a part of the food supply into the food. Like they're trying to make a corn so that is resistant to certain pests, insects and other plant life. So they're using pesticides like D-Aspartic that ultimately becomes Agent Orange. That's being used to breed into the corn, so that the corn can resist these other pests. But D-Aspartic's also poisonous to humans. The trouble that our troops have had in Vietnam with Agent Orange is proof of that.

Another related product is the Roundup chemical from Monsanto which has long been considered hazardous to humans. It's being bred into the corn. How long can we make these products a part of the corn before they infect us? And how long can we feed this corn to animals, before the animals become pesticides? And we become pesticides.

This is common knowledge, this is nothing new from me. But the companies that make these chemicals originally made them to be used in germ warfare in World War I. And they modify the D'Aspartic to try and protect their own bottom line. But it's basically the same thing that's being bred into corn, canola-- products that I am avoiding more and more when I buy my groceries.

One change I've seen in the past few decades has been the consumer preference for lower fat milk as opposed to whole milk. Whole milk is about 3¾ or 3½% butterfat. Skim milk has none and you can buy 1%, 2% also. But when you separate fat from the milk, you know the fat globules in the milk, microscopic in size, that little segment of fat is surrounded by a molecule thick layer of protein. So when you remove the fat from the milk, you're also removing the protein. When you homogenize milk, you're breaking down this protein shell so the fat mixes in with the milk and you can't separate it. Therefore, the skim milk has to be processed before these little particles are broken down. Therefore the protein is also taken out when you let the fat rise to the top and you just skim it off. That's why it's called skim milk. Once you homogenize the milk, that can't happen. So when you're making skim milk, you're making a milk product that's very devoid of protein. And skim milk naturally has a blueish tint to it, which the consumers are not too crazy about. They're not used to seeing milk that is blue. And I can understand that. And as a way around this, the dairies add a casein product that was taken out of the milk when making other products. But when they put this casein back in, from what I understand, the pasteurization is done afterwards and this casein product can become, DOES become, carcinogenic.

Farmer Rob Moutoux   Interviewed 6/4/14

Rob Moutoux: My name is Rob Moutoux and we're here at Moutoux Orchard. We're in Purcellville, VA, and we grow fruit trees. Historically, that's been our main crop. But we now operate what we call a whole diet year-round CSA program. So we offer pasture-raised meats, vegetables, pasture-raised unpasteurized dairy. That's sort of a mouthful. And then eggs, and also some whole grains to our CSA membership of about 40 households. And we operate year round. Our family's been in business for about 65 years and we've been offering the whole diet CSA program for about four years now.

I have done a lot of different grains. We've grown wheat, spelt, rye, oats and barley-- all cereal grains. And at this point we're only growing wheat for human consumption. It's a soft red winter wheat. It's historically what grows best around here. And we don't use any pesticides. We don't use any herbicides or fertilizer, commercial/conventional fertilizer on the grains. And we mill our own flour for the membership.

Tamar: Are they called organic grains or is that not a--

Rob: We don't buy certified organic seed, but we save our own seed. At some point I bought conventional seed but we have been saving a strain of seed for several years now. And again it's a soft red winter wheat. But, I guess at this point three years afterwards, it would be, you know, if we were certified, organic. It would be certifiable.

Tamar: Is there any issue with the government at all, the fact that you have your own seed?

Rob: No. No. 'Cause it's not patented seed. It wasn't GMO to start with. So it's not a patented seed that I'm saving. It's just, you know, it was conventionally grown but no patents on the seed. So it's my option to choose to save that, which is good.

Tamar: Can you sell that anywhere, or does it have to be locally?

Rob: Well, we don't have a major market for it, so in the past I've sold flour at the farmers markets. I'm not doing that anymore. So we only sell our grains and flour through the CSA program. So we don't go off the farm to do any distributing. So it's a pretty small scale.

Tamar: What is the difference between GMO and non-GMO, for grains?

Rob: GMO stands for Genetically Modified Organisms. There are a lot of claims that are made about negative impacts to human health, and livestock health, from eating GMO crops. And they're, the studies and the claims, are such that we just want to avoid GMO crops and we want to raise our crops non-GMO. And we also aren't using the pesticides, so if you were marketing yourself as organic, you can't use GMO crops or seed. And that's by the book.

Tamar: What made you choose specifically not to do that?

Rob: I'm just a believer in good, good health. And I like feeding good food, and we really focus on good soil. And definitely believe that good soil, mineral-rich, biologically-active, all the good stuff promotes good food and good health, both for livestock and for humans. And that's why I believe in it.

Tamar: Do you think that, and I know all this is just your opinion, but do you think that anything that is fed to the livestock should be included perhaps in the labeling of the food that you purchase?

Rob: It's important for consumers to realize that when they're eating animal products, they're also eating everything that that animal ate. And that means if it's not organic, it very well, and most certainly is, a GMO crop. And so it's important if you're going to eat animal products and you're trying to avoid GMO, then you need to avoid non-organic animal products.

I feel like, the best thing that I can say for a consumer that's looking to get this type of food is to start having a conversation with the people that are growing the food. And really, that's where it starts. So there are a lot of questions to be asked, and there are a lot of different opinions, and a lot of people saying one thing or another thing, and there are a lot of labels. But when you have that intimate conversation with the consumer to the grower, it sort of goes beyond the labels. And, you know, the person buying the food can get a feel for, "Is this person growing food? And is this the type of person that is gonna grow the food that I want to be eating?" I think ultimately that's where a lot of it comes from. But, at the same time, don't just buy into the fact that this is local food, therefore it's good food, because that's not always true. You know, it really depends on farm to farm to farm.

Tamar: Do you think it's something in the pasteurization process that's making people sick?

Rob: It's not necessarily making people sick, it might mean that they're missing out on some of the goodies also, as in the good bacteria-- that sort of being damaged through pasteurization has a huge impact on our gut flora and therefore our overall states of health and potentially to allergies. But anecdotally, we definitely hear things like that from our members, things like, you know, "Our son has allergies and we've been on the raw milk, and now he doesn't," or, "They're diminished." Even things like allergies to cats, you know, those have been diminished through drinking raw milk.

Tamar: What about milk allergies? Are-- I mean, are people, some people able to drink raw milk that couldn't drink regular?

Rob: Anecdotally, from what our members tell us, raw milk has been very, very helpful for allergies. And so, that's a nice thing. The fairly standard view is that a lactose intolerance-- people that are lactose intolerant can drink raw milk because there's lactase enzymes in the raw milk. Whereas in pasteurized milk those enzymes are damaged and destroyed. And so obviously the enzyme that's meant to break down that milk protein, if it's not there, then you're gonna have problems digesting them if you can't make them yourself and I think that's the issue. So, if you can't make them yourselves and you're drinking milk and there is the enzyme that's meant to digest what you're drinking, then it makes more sense that people don't have the problem with raw milk. And that's something that I hear fairly often from our members.

Tamar: Jack, just tell me your name and where we are, a little bit about the farm.

Jack Lazor: Okay. I'm Jack Lazor and this is Butterworks Farm here in Westfield, Vermont. We're right on the Canadian border and we've been here since 1976. And we've built a farm organism on our farm here. So we have Jersey cows, we process dairy products. We grow hay for them, and we grow grain for them, although less and less grain for them, and more and more grain for people. I grow a variety of organic grains. Probably my wheat is my biggest crop for flour production-- and barley, oats, some peas once in a while. I've grown flax. And then I grow some corn and soybeans. And these are all in rotation with hay crops. And the corn and soybeans, well, we also grow seed, too. I process a lot of grain seed, you know, with this cleaner that's right over here. And we also clean all of our human consumption grain. As far as finances go, it's a small part of our operation. Mostly processing milk into dairy products is our major income generator, but this is really my passion right here, is growing grains. And then we produce the straw, and then we use the straw to bed the cows in basically a big bedding pack. And it's six feet thick come spring and then the compost is out on the main road out there. It's all turned into compost and then it goes back to the land, here, on the farm. So grain, the straw that we get from the grain sometimes is almost as important as the grain itself.

Tamar: So, if the only way to eat is to find organic, what are our options?

Jack: The options for people out there are to know your farmer, first and foremost. Buy local. Go to the farmers market and establish relationships with producers. So what this takes, is this takes a lot more effort than people are accustomed to, to buy their food. And, you know, some people are going to want to do this, and some people aren't, depending on how passionate you are about what you eat. And unfortunately, there's still a rather large proportion of our country here that doesn't really want to make the effort to really know what they're eating. They're more interested in riding their four-wheeler or watching their show on TV tonight. So that's the rub right there. You will have to pay more. And you will have to care. And I think, the one thing I can see changing is that this GMO experiment that they've sort of rammed down our throat for the last 20 years, as it manifests itself in our population and people keep getting immune system problems and food allergies, gradually we'll wake up to the fact that this was not such a good thing.

And if the Europeans can pay between 20 and 30% of their annual salary to eat really, really good food, we can go from 8% in this country up to 14 or 15 and I think we'd be a whole lot better off for it.

Jack and Anne Lazor are the creators and founders of Butterworks Farm. They came to Westfield in 1976 fresh out of college with degrees in Agricultural History (Jack) and Anthropology (Anne). As longtime sustainable farmers and leaders in organic farming they continue to

[99]

play an important role in the dynamics and operations at Butterworks and beyond. Jack is a writer and frequent inspirational keynote speaker at organic farming conferences everywhere. He enjoys food, friends and pursuing his passions- sustainability and soil science. Anne keeps Jack and the farm running as Jack's home dialysis technician and a caring presence for the entire team. She enjoys gardening, keeping chickens and ducks, the study of homeopathic medicine and upholds the homesteading spirit she and Jack started with 40 years ago. (http://butterworksfarm.com)

Jack is the author of The Organic Grain Grower.

Michael: Name is Mike Snow. We are in Leesburg, VA. I have a farm. Willowsford Farm. Where I grow vegetables, mixed vegetables. We raise goats. We sell honey. We sell all sorts of goods at the farm stands.

Tamar: Okay. So you were telling me the other day that this is not a certified organic farm, but that you do things in an organic way. What does it mean to be organic or not organic and what do you do differently?

Michael: There's a lot of different ways to farm. As farmers we all have to deal with the same issues, if it's weeds, if it's insect pests, if it's other kinds of pests, diseases, things like this. So when we talk about organic or when we talk about conventional, part of what we're talking about is how are we managing our crops. How are we managing our vegetables? In that how do we respond to all the different stresses that happen? So, I mean, there's so much that we can't control. But then the question is, well, what do you do about it? As an organic farmer, or whether or not we're certified, we're looking for cultural practices and biological responses, rather than chemical responses.

So, the conventional farmer, if they see that they tend to get a disease on their tomato plants, are more likely to use chemistry/chemicals to fumigate, to kill the pathogen. As organic farmers, we might do a bunch of things. Sort of, "many little hammers," we talk about. So we'll use cultural practices like proper spacing between plants. We raise the plants off the ground so that-- we orient them with the wind so that winds will dry them off, less likely to get fungal diseases. And then, if we have to, we would use either sort of a probiotic type of an approach on our plants. So, encouraging the good microorganisms on the leaf or on the plant so that they'll out-compete the bad ones.

And other times, if we sort of need to rescue something, then we might. And if we do that, then we would use something that's organically approved. Meaning either it comes from-- it's sort of a natural ingredient, or it's something that breaks down very quickly. But as a general rule we use things that aren't going be toxic to the environment, aren't going be toxic to us. In part, just because I don't like to spray those things. I don't want to do that kind of work.

So whether or not we're certified organic the certification process is really about the relationship you have with your customers. So, if I'm selling wholesale then I don't know my customers, they don't know me. And so, by having someone else than the federal government or the agencies that represent the government certification process, they kind of stand-in for that relationship.

So that if you go to the store and you want to buy tomatoes that I happen to grow, you can know, because they are certified organic, that they were grown in a certain way. Whereas I sell almost all of my product direct to our community members and direct to our customers. They know me, I know them. They can see the farm. We invite them to our farm.

We talk about what we do. There's really no secrets on our farm. So, that certification process isn't really necessary.

Tamar: Is there anything that you would need to change about how you do something to make you certified?

Michael: There's one thing that we do. We use a biodegradable mulch for some of our crops. And this is, the material is certified for organic use in Europe and in Canada, and supposedly it's under review for the United States. But right now the way the certification process works in the U.S., you can't use the biodegradable mulch.

And so until they can show that it fits the organic standards, then, it's not. Instead, we'd have to use black plastic which is a petroleum product. And then we'd have to pull it up every year. Whereas, to me, it's more important, I'd have to throw that out. And it's a petroleum product. And, you know, you can't get away from that entirely, but it's not something we like to use.

Whereas with the biodegradable mulch, we put it in and we mulch around it with straw. And then when we're done with the crop, that stuff breaks down in the soil so it just acts as a fertilizer. That's the only thing we do.

Tamar: What are we doing now in farming that we weren't doing many years ago? What is the difference in our food supply in general?

Michael: I'm not a farm historian. But I think that you can sort of look at the way that agriculture's evolved in the last, well in the last 10,000 years in a sense, but especially in the last several hundred years-- in the last maybe 100/150/200 years actually. We've been able to mechanize a lot of things. So, as we've started to build tractors-- that might be the most important thing. We found that we can, instead of using animal power or human power to till up the soil, to dig the soil, to dig weeds, once that mechanical traction came in, we didn't need the animals anymore.

And so suddenly you've divorced two parts of agriculture, the animal agriculture and the plant agriculture. Whereas before you had animals and so they would-- manure-- and you would grow crops for them to eat and then they would. So you'd sort of create this rotation. But especially the manure, which would then get turned back into the ground.

And once we started using mechanical traction, we don't need those anymore. And so you can have just a crop, just a crop system or just an animal system. And so suddenly you're looking for new kinds of efficiencies when you do that. That's probably the biggest change.

And being able to do more. With a tractor you can dig up more ground. You can dig deeper. You can till both in volume and in depth. And that causes a lot more soil damage. And so we've exacerbated the problems that we've been able to mitigate because we haven't had that kind of power.

Tamar: I assume you prefer eating food from your own farm.

Michael: Yes.

Tamar: What scares you about conventional food or other farms? What makes you stick to your own?

Michael: There's a couple answers. I mean, there's sort of me as a consumer-- I don't know what I don't know. Right? Like, when you buy in a grocery store there's no face on it. There's no relationship. But it's less of what I'm afraid of, or worried about from other food. I mean, you sort of assume that there's gonna be some pesticide residue or something like that on food that you find in the grocery store. I know there's none of that on my food, because that's not how I roll. But more, it's that I know how I feel when I eat a plant, or a leaf of a plant that's alive. I see it. I take it. I graze during the day. When I go home at night, I just say, "You know the chard looks great. I'm going to take some of this Swiss chard." Or I pull some garlic out of the ground. It's still alive. It's still respiring. And you get a different kind of energy when you buy something, even the same Swiss chard at the store. It just isn't quite as lively or as fresh. That's the difference.

Tamar: Can you explain what genetically modified is?

Michael: We select for whatever traits we want. But it's always been done within the ancestral genetics of that species. There's never been a crossing between, say, wheat and a tomato, because that's impossible. Or differently, we've certainly never crossed a plant with a fish, or with a mouse, or whatever it might be.

[105]

Or a bacteria. Because we've never been able to do that. We've never had the technology for that.

There are different strategies for breeding within plants. And certainly we've started to hybridize plants, where we'll take a corn, this kind of corn and this kind of corn, and we'll put them together in the lab, where they might not naturally have crossed. And that's sort of the modern hybridization process.

Genetic engineering is a new thing, where we're able to splice genes from one species, of all of the species on the planet, and splice that into another species. So completely different kingdoms even. That's something that wouldn't be able to happen without us, or, without certain viruses that are used to actually transfer the genetics from the one species to the other. That's sort of the difference between genetic engineering and any kind of traditional plant breeding.

Tamar: You told me how each farmer has to pick and choose whatever trait you want the most. So how do you pick and choose? Is there a "right" way?

Michael: Well, seed selection is part philosophy, it's part economics, it's part what your customers want. We grow-- because we sell direct and we sell local and we sell fresh-- the things that are important to us and they're important to our customers. And so we don't make the same decisions that a farmer who is wholesaling out of California or out of Arizona, or even out of another part of Virginia, makes.

So what we're looking for are varieties that look and taste great. We're looking for varieties that grow well under our conditions which in the mid-Atlantic are challenging. I mean it's very humid here. It gets very hot, and then it gets very cold, or the vice-versa. We want varieties that grow well in our soils and respond well to our cultural practices. So as an organic farmer, I would prefer a variety that's not used to getting high doses of chemical fertilizers or soluble salt fertilizers.

Whereas an organic variety, often is going to be sort of more thrifty in the soil, be able to get what it wants. Quality-wise we're talking about taste, which often has to do with the same soil/plant interaction. And we're also talking about the phytochemical content. So the more nutrition in a variety, often that translates into taste.

The opposite of that would be, if I were selling wholesale tomatoes to ship across the country so that they're available on the other coast, whatever, wherever, however far away it is, so that they're available at a time of year where they otherwise aren't available. Meaning-- Mexico or California can grow tomatoes through the winter whereas I can't grow them here without high inputs of heat.

I'm looking for something else. I'm looking for something that I can pick early, and something that has a standard look. Because people buy based on their eyes. And we have learned to think that a tomato should be perfectly round, and very red, with that little bit of green on top, and perfectly blemish-free, of course, too.

Also looking for something that's going to stand up to the shipping. So no matter how much packaging we've kind of-- how much we've softened the trip, a tomato's going to be in a truck for several days, at the least. It's going to be in a grocery store for a while, but first it's in a warehouse. It's moving around a lot. And it's sort of enduring that.

So when the person is breeding a tomato that can take all of that transport and then still last on the shelf for at least 5 days or something, you're breeding for characteristics that generally aren't going to taste good.

The largest vegetable seed company in the world was bought in the last several years by Monsanto. They're not the only company. And that's what companies do. But, but it certainly raises alarms. I mean you certainly see fewer and fewer people-- PEOPLE, not just the COMPANY-- but fewer people/decision makers, having control over what seeds and what genetics are available.

I know that there's a lot of question about what can be patented now. But my fear is that if we, as farmers, rely on seed that is owned by just a few people, then we have less to offer our customers, our community. In my case at least, directly, my community are my customers. I have less options of what to grow. Not to envision some dystopian universe but, there's certainly the possibilities that maybe a genetically engineered crop is the only option. The likelihood of that happening is pretty miniscule. But we just don't know. We don't have control.

The alternative universe to that is one in which seeds, especially germ plasm, is sort of an open source, piece of information-- where the people who breed plants have access to all sorts of germ plasm and can breed all sorts of different crops for different conditions, for different tastes, for different colors, for different shipping abilities-- and where there wouldn't be that kind of control and ownership over that.

We grow a lot of open-pollinated varieties because I think that they tend to taste better. I can eat them fresher. They look more interesting. People seem to like them. I like growing them. But we also grow hybrids because maybe they taste better. It would be very upsetting to me, and I think to a lot of my customers, if we lost those varieties.

Tamar: Do we start to label every ingredient in the feed of animals just to include everything?

Michael: Maybe that is the most appropriate thing to do. If people find they are sensitive to corn-fed beef or corn-fed chicken, then they have a right to know what they're eating. Otherwise, it's on them to find out. And we get those questions. We get people looking for, "Is there soy in your feed?" Yes, right now, there's soy in our feed. If more people say they want soy-free feed for the chickens, then I'm happy to raise them on it. It costs us a lot more and we're going to have to pass that cost on. If people are willing to pay for it, I'm glad to do it. I don't have a problem with that.

Tamar: That's why it pays to know your farmer.

Michael: Well, that's right.

Tamar: You can ask the questions.

Michael: If regulations are not going to do this thing for us, then it's on us to do that. And the only way you're going to find out, it will be easiest for you if you can go up to the farmer and ask. I mean, it's a lot harder to get through a company to find out for sure.

Tamar: Are you for or against GMO? Or is it a grey area?

Michael: I see why people use GE crops. It doesn't jive with my philosophy in farming, or maybe in life, too. Obviously they're sort of connected. As far as I can tell, if you're growing crops in a more ecological manner, then the need for a genetically engineered crop, I don't know that it exists.

There are different reasons for using genetically engineered crops. Some genetically engineered crops are designed to resist a certain pathogen, like mangos or bananas. Something like that. Others are modified so that they will be resistant to herbicide. So corn and soy might be Roundup Ready meaning, you can grow your corn and you can let the weeds go, you can dump the herbicide on it. The herbicide would otherwise damage the corn, but this corn is designed to resist that damage, so it kills everything except the corn. The corn is the last man standing on that field.

Another type of genetically engineered crop is one that has an insecticide as part of its genetics. So if an army worm, or a corn ear worm, or a looper or a monarch butterfly-- I mean, that's sort of the scary part, the collateral damage-- if it eats any part of the plant it'll die, because it'll ingest the toxin. I don't have the need for that, in part, because I grow things in a polyculture as much as possible, meaning, I don't grow 100 acres of one thing. If anything, I grow many

[110]

crops very close together. I rotate them so that they're constantly sort of outrunning pests, or trying to.

We often grow insectary strips. We often grow living mulches or non-living mulches so that pests will have a hard time finding our crops. There're a lot of things that we can do as farmers to avoid the need for something like that. So to me it's like, "Why would I use that when I have other cultural practices that negate the need for it?"

An insect generally is attracted to the same things that indicate that a plant is unhealthy. So basically when they're looking, they're seeing sort of the colors of an unhealthy plant, and that's attractive to them. So they're like, "All right I'm gonna chow down." So by raising a healthy plant, we actually minimize a lot of our crop damage. You know, it's not a perfect situation. Not all of our pests are insects, of course. But we certainly find that the healthier our crops are, then the less likely they are to get fungal diseases, bacteria diseases, insect damage. That relates directly with the nutritional content. I mean a healthy plant, right, it's going to have healthy food. Healthy food produces the part of the plant that we eat, is going to have a higher nutritional content, too. So that's where we get into the consumption side and whether or not we are eating food that's healthy for us.

So just because you've got a bunch of collards at the store, doesn't mean that they're going to be of the highest quality. We know that for the last 75 years or so, from studies started by the USDA, that the nutritional content of foods, of raw vegetables, is not what it used to be. So, a carrot that's taken off the shelf analyzed for major nutrients and major vitamins, now, on average shows maybe a quarter to a half of the nutritional content that it used to. And that's sort of a common theme. Whether it's always that percent, I don't know. But, what does that mean? That means you have to eat four times as many carrots. Who's going to do that? But we think that by raising a crop that's healthier in the first place and that where we focus on making sure that it has the proper nutrition, that we have a higher quality product, make people feel better they don't have to eat as much to feel full and physically satisfied. Becomes a quality issue.

http://willowsford.com/farm-conservancy

Falko: My name is Falko Schilling and I'm the
consumer protection advocate for Vermont Public
Interest Research Group. VPIRG is the state's largest
non-profit consumer environmental advocacy group.
We have over 30,000 members and supporters over
the state of Vermont. We advocate on a wide range of
issues including GMO labeling as well as fighting
carbon pollution and also try to protect Vermonters
from toxic chemicals.

Tamar: Why are GMOs not listed on packaging?

Falko: GMOs are not listed on packaging here in the
U.S. because there are large special interests that
have fought tooth and nail to make sure that they are
not. We've seen this in California. We saw it in
Washington, where we had two of the biggest ballot
initiatives in terms of spending, where large
companies came in and dumped millions of dollars
against giving consumers the right to know what's in
their food. And this is just an example of what's been
happening on the federal level trying to make sure
what happened in Europe, where consumers were
given this information, doesn't happen here in the
U.S.

Tamar: Is it important for GMOs to be listed on
packaging?

Falko: I think it's extremely important for GMOs to be
listed on food packaging for a number of reasons.
Consumers from all walks of life are asking for this

[113]

information and that's the job of the government to make sure that this information is given to consumers because they think it's material and they think it makes a difference in their daily lives.

Tamar: What exactly are you fighting for in terms of labeling right at this moment?

Falko: So what we're fighting for at this moment is that we're trying to make sure that the federal courts uphold Vermonters' right to know what's in their food and make sure that the courts keep in place Vermont's first-in-the-nation, no-strings-attached GMO labeling bill. This is a first-in-the-nation law in terms of its effects. And because of that, we've brought down a lot of, shall we say, anger from some of the larger food manufacturers and other industries that don't want to see state-based labeling and honestly don't want to see federal labeling of genetically engineered food as well. So they've taken the State of Vermont to court to try and make sure that this law is thrown out and Vermonters don't know what's in their food.

Tamar: What would you like to see on the labels, and why is it important to you?

Falko: Well, one thing I'd definitely would like to see on labels is the fact of whether or not a food is genetically engineered. This is something that has been kept in the dark from consumers for a long time and it's something that we need more information about. I think there's a number of other issues that we can try and make sure that information is on the label but this is something consumers have been calling for

for almost 20 years. And it's now just taking hold in the United States and I'm very happy Vermont is taking the lead on making sure consumers have this information.

Tamar: What is the biggest challenge that we have right now?

Falko: Generally from the food system perspective, I think there's a lot of challenges. The biggest one, I would say, right now, is education. People need to find out where their food's coming from, how it's grown. And that's what's really driving a lot of this consumer demand for more information. They want to know where it comes from, if pesticides are used. And especially, they want to know if their food is genetically engineered.

Tamar: Why is it that ingredients listed on food labels don't begin to explain what's actually in each component of an ingredient? I mean, how did something like "natural flavoring" ever end up in a package? What does that even mean?

Falko: So "natural flavoring" is one of those things that I don't think means a whole lot. Just like when you see a bag of potato chips that tells you it's natural, that means very, very little. And this all because the federal government has a loose regulatory scheme saying what you can actually put on a package. And we're starting to see a lot more pushback around that, especially on things like "natural" where folks have been making that claim, in my opinion, falsely for a number of years, saying that foods that are by definition, not natural, could be labeled as such in a grocery store.

Tamar: So do you think this is a state by state issue or it's a national issue, or both?

Falko: Well, I think it's a national issue, I think it's an international issue, but that we're not seeing any action on a federal level right now, particularly because of all the large special interests such as Monsanto and the major food manufacturers that don't want to see a federal standard. Because of that, I think this is something that needs to happen at the state level. People in states like Vermont, and Oregon, and Colorado need to stand up and say, "We want to see these foods labeled," before we're actually going to see any action on a federal level.

Tamar: What would surprise us to learn? What do you know that we don't know?

Falko: Well. I don't really know much that I think the general public doesn't know too much about. It might surprise people to know just what percentage of the food grown in the United States is actually genetically engineered. You look at the percentage of corn, cotton, soy, canola, sugar beets. Those are things that increasingly are becoming genetically engineered. And it's either going into processed foods or it's going into animal feed. And I guess maybe one thing I would add that people, a lot of people don't know and would be surprised about is, when you see on an ingredient label that it says something's made out of sugar, a lot of time it's coming from a beet. It's a lot of times coming from a genetically engineered beet. So unless you see it says "cane sugar," you don't really have that information. So that might be something that surprises folks.

Tamar: What are they trying to keep a secret?

Falko: Well, I think one of the biggest reasons that food companies are trying to keep this information off of food labels-- 'cause they're afraid about protecting their profits. They've built a system around using genetically engineered foods without telling consumers about it and they're afraid there's going to be consumer backlash when they find out what's actually in their foods. And they don't want to disrupt the way that they're doing business.

I think that if you look at the amount of corn produced in the United States, it's something that is making its way into our food in a number of different ways, from corn syrup to all kinds of other ingredients that are highly processed that people just wouldn't expect are being made out of corn. It's become our new sugar and because it's cheap and we can produce a heck of a lot of it. And Americans have an undying desire for sugar.

Tamar: Is there anything else in general that you would like to say?

Falko: Well I think what I would say is that for folks all across the country who are working to try and make sure that their food is labeled properly, that if it can happen in Vermont, then it can happen across the country. And whether it's going to the ballot box to make it happen, or working with your legislature, you can make it happen. It just takes mobilization. It takes

[117]

working with people in your community and making sure they are feeling comfortable to raise their voice on these issues.

Falko Schilling, Esq. has worked in Vermont State House on a wide range of issues including health care reform, consumer protection, and environmental regulation since 2010. A native of Vermont, Falko received his law degree from Vermont Law School and is a licensed attorney. Before joining Action Circles, Falko spent five years leading winning legislative and grassroots campaigns as the Consumer and Environmental Advocate at Vermont Public Interest Research Group. Major victories included helping pass the nation's first mandatory genetically engineered food labeling law, and allowing dental therapists to practice in Vermont. (linkedin.com)

Linda: My name is Linda B. Rosenthal. I'm New York State Assembly member, representing the 67th Assembly District, which is Upper West Side and parts of Clinton/Hell's Kitchen.

Tamar: Okay. So this is a quote from your bill. "Currently there's no federal law that requires food producers to identify whether foods were produced with genetic engineering," and the FDA does not require safety studies of these foods. So is that still the case?

Linda: Yes. That's absolutely still the case. Currently, and for a while, despite pressure from various advocacy groups, the FDA has declined to wade into the GMO labeling fight. And they've decided, you know, they don't need to evaluate studies to see if GMOs are safe or even require studies. So they've decided, for the time being, not to require any kind of labeling on GMOs.

Tamar: Also from your bill, "More than 60 countries including key United States trading partners have laws mandating disclosure of genetically engineered foods. So identifying foods produced with genetic engineering will protect our state's export market."

Linda: The ironic thing is that, when food manufacturers in the States send food abroad to Italy or China, or other countries that do not accept GMOs or require GMO labeling, they have to do that on the foods they (export). Yet, they maintain that it is a burden to do it for people eating and living in the United States. And that's totally unacceptable.

Tamar: Why do you think we're so behind the rest of the world?

Linda: Well, in this country, and I'm sure in other countries, but in this country, big business, big corporations often just rule the roost. And we can see by the amount of millions that Monsanto and Pepsi and the Grocery Manufacturers' Association have piled into campaigns against GMO labeling efforts across the country, they don't want it. They do not want labeling. They're willing to spend millions and millions to prevent labeling and so they're winning the day, at this moment.

Tamar: Also from your bill, "Without disclosure, consumers with certain dietary restrictions may unknowingly consume such food in violation of dietary restrictions."

Linda: One of the reasons that so many people want products with genetic engineering labeled, is because they do not want to consume those kinds of foods, whether it's the chemicals in the grain that gets sprayed with glyphosate or other herbicides. I know some women who've recently had babies and they say, "I want to feed my baby everything organic or safe for them." And they don't know which foods to avoid, which have GMOs and which do not right now, because there's no labeling.

I mean, you can conjecture, you can guess, you can try to stay away from certain foods, but why shouldn't it be easy for the consumer to just see, "Oh this has a

GMO in it, I'm gonna stay away"? Or for those who don't care, doesn't matter. The label's there, doesn't matter. But for those who wish to avoid it for health reasons, or any other reason, they should have that right. They're spending their money on the product.

Tamar: What is your biggest challenge in this fight?

Linda: In my view, the biggest challenge is fighting the corporate giants who are dedicated to ensuring that no foods will be labeled in the United States. And by corporate giants, I mean companies like Dow and DuPont, Monsanto, Pepsi Cola. You know, most of the big corporate manufacturers use genetic engineering and so they don't want to have to label anything.

And they have come up with a host of reasons from, "it'll cost too much," which, you know, they change labels all the time to say "new" and "light" and "low calorie." I mean, that is a specious argument. But they go from that to "labels signify something bad." "So if you label something, it would dissuade a consumer from purchasing it," which is also nonsense, because we have a lot of information on labels right now, especially with the new requirements to have larger type and to talk about the sugars in there, that the federal government has mandated now. So the fact that they don't want labeling means that every effort in every state is challenged. And they overwhelm the local media. They do mailings, they have ads on TV, they have social media. And places, for example, like California, which at first polling, people were like, "Yes, we want to label GMOs," after millions were spent, they ended up rejecting the referendum.

So it's hard to compete against these well-funded opposition. And so the pro GMO (labeling) people have to raise more money. We're never going to have the same amount of money, but we have to try to compete with them in certain ways, like in media. I don't know any activists who doesn't want labeling. So, we have the people-- it's just their ability to move money into different states to broadcast.

At the same time though, a number of states, not through referendum but through the legislature, have passed GMO labeling bills, for example, Connecticut, Maine, Vermont. And in those, some of those states, the big corporate giants are suing to prevent the labeling from going into effect.

Tamar: Do you think this is a state by state issue? Or a national issue?

Linda: Ideally, this would be a purely national issue where the federal government, the Congress would pass a law mandating that all foods containing GMOs be so labeled. However, it's not going that way. So the alternate way of going about this is to do this campaign state by state. And when you reach critical mass then the federal government will look and say, "You know what? We really need to codify this nationwide." So that's the strategy right now.

Tamar: So what would surprise us to learn? What do you know that we don't know yet?

Linda: I think people in general are not clued in about the amount of money behind the effort to block labeling of GMOs. So for example, Grocery Manufacturers Association -- there was a case in

California, that the attorney general is investigating, where Pepsi and Monsanto, and Dow and DuPont, and many other companies, funneled contributions through the Grocery Manufacturers Association. So they didn't have to be public about them, to oppose the referendum.

And if people knew how much was being put into the fight against labeling, and convincing, actually manipulating people to think that it's unnecessary and maybe a bad thing to label, I think they'd look a little further into if it's to just label or not label. What is the reason behind trying to block it? What is the reason for pouring millions of dollars into the effort to block it? It's certainly not about the consumer. It's about the business people, their bottom line and their need to keep profits over people's health and people's right to know.

Assembly member Linda B. Rosenthal represents the 67th Assembly district, which includes the Upper West Side and parts of Clinton/Hell's Kitchen in Manhattan. Elected in 2006 after serving for 13 years as Manhattan District Director and Director of Special Projects for United States Congressman Jerrold Nadler, Rosenthal succeeded then – Assembly member, now New York City Comptroller Scott M. Stringer.

Since then, Assembly member Rosenthal has passed more than 70 laws that have helped to improve the lives of all New York State residents. In previous sessions, Rosenthal has passed laws extending orders of protection to companion animals whose abuse often serves as a warning sign; requiring that applicants of public assistance be provided with information and resources for victims of sexual assault; allowing for same sex couples to adopt non-biological children together in New York State; and prohibiting the sale of electronic cigarettes to minors. In her tenure, Rosenthal has established herself as a leading advocate on affordable housing, domestic violence, consumer protection, government reform, environmental issues and animal cruelty.

Assembly member Rosenthal received a B.A. in History from the University of Rochester. She is a lifelong resident of the Upper West Side.

Chair, Committee on Alcoholism and Drug Abuse. Standing Committee Assignments: Agriculture; Alcoholism and Drug Abuse, Corporations, Authorities and Commissions; Energy; Housing; Health; Tourism, Parks, Arts and Sports. (http://nyassembly.gov/mem/Linda-B-Rosenthal/bio/)

Tamar: Hello. Just introduce yourself.

Patty: Patty Lovera, and we're at Food and Water Watch in Washington, DC. I'm the assistant director and I run our food policy program.

So Food and Water Watch is a consumer advocacy organization and we really work on trying to educate people about what's going on in the food supply, but also get them involved. So, we want people to know what they're buying and do a better job with that, but we also want people to get involved to change the food system. It's a political issue.

Tamar: What current projects are you working on?

Patty: So we do a lot of work on the rules for safety. We have a very strong system historically for the safety of meat and poultry. We have government inspectors in those plants, looking at those products, and there's always attacks on that system. So we've been in a fight for many, many years. And it's really hot right now-- there's a proposal to cut government inspection of chicken and let the companies do more inspection themselves. So we spend a ton of time on that. We think that's a terrible idea.

We do spend a lot of time on GMO issues, both trying to stop new approvals-- so there's a bunch, there's always new, new crops that the biotech industry wants to get on the market, new GMO crops-- a whole push for 2,4-D ready crops, a GMO potato, genetically engineered salmon-- we're working on all those, but we're also working usually at a state level, closer to the grass roots. There's a lot of activity trying to get labeling of these foods, so we're real involved in that issue too.

Tamar: What do you want to see on the labels? What's important to get on the labels?

Patty: So we think labeling is the bare minimum that people can, or that companies could do. I mean there's a lot of controversies about how we're raising our food. It has changed pretty dramatically in a short period of time. We're doing a lot of things differently than we used to. And the rules aren't strong enough. The science isn't good enough to really understand what we're doing. So there's a lot we need to fix, but at a minimum we should be telling people what they're eating so they can decide for themselves. So we think labeling is just the first step to really tackling a lot of the things we're concerned about, a lot of the questions that we have.

I mean at this point, we're asking for a really reasonable thing, and it's astonishing how much the industry hates it. And that's just, I'll never get over how much they're opposed to what's really a common sense requirement that says "produced with genetic engineering" or "contains genetically engineered ingredients." That's it. It's not a warning label. It's not anything more than that. It doesn't mess with the nutrition effects box. It doesn't mess with the ingredient list. It's just that disclosure.

Pretty basic. A couple of words. And they are fighting this tooth and nail because they don't want people to know this most basic piece of information about how this food was produced. That's all we're asking for. It's pretty basic. And it's pretty hard to argue with. I mean you go to the public, people are like, "Of course I should have that. Why shouldn't I get to know this about my food?" It's just really these companies that don't want people to have really any idea what's going on.

Tamar: What are your concerns about GMOs?

Patty: So we have a lot of concerns about GMOs. They range from big picture, you know, "What are they doing to the food supply, what are they doing to the economics and the ownership and the control of the food supply," and then we're really concerned that we don't know enough about whether they're safe to eat. And the regulations and the system we have for proving them is really weak. For all this talk from the biotech industry about how regulated they are, they're really not very regulated at all. They do the science and give that data to the government, which doesn't do their own science.

You know, we have very little independent research. And we don't even get to track what's happening to people who eat these foods because we don't tell people they're eating these foods because we don't label them. So then there's environmental concerns. I mean, this is a technology that's very closely tied to chemical use in the fields. There's environmental impacts from that. There's public health impacts from that. So it's just, at every layer kinda from macro to personal consumption we have concerns.

Tamar: What would surprise us to learn?

Patty: Oh boy. Oh, I have so many things! Let me pick. I think for the GMO issue, I think lots of consumers are really shocked to understand what it is, like what the actual technology is and who benefits from it. 'Cause it's not consumers and it's actually not really farmers. It's these seed companies. And they're seed companies who were actually chemical companies first. Right?

And so I think that the link is real. It's very hard to break the link between GMOs as they're being mostly used at this point. And these chemical companies are changing these crops so that they can be exposed to pretty tough chemicals, and that they'll survive and the weeds are supposed to die. And now it's not working. We've so overused these chemicals that the weeds are now resistant to the first generation. And we're moving onto a next generation. And we're talking about tougher chemicals.

So the next generation of GMO crops is going to be packaged up to work with 2,4-D. 2,4-D was an ingredient in Agent Orange. It is a tough chemical that's tough on the environment, on farm workers, on public health. We shouldn't be using more of it. And that's what gonna happen if we go this route, and use more. So I think that it just really goes against all of the marketing and the PR and the hype that we hear from Monsanto and from these companies about feeding the world and fixing the environment.

This is about selling their chemicals. That's why they started to package them and change these seeds. I think the business model is what I think shocks a lot of consumers. And then the other big thing I think is the extent-- I think consumers are shocked when they kind of get a little exposure to the fight over labeling in particular, and they realize the extent to which these companies do not want this information out there. The millions of, tens of millions of dollars that are being spent to prevent this minor change, this minor requirement that you just say, we use this technology, that's it? They're spending tens of millions of dollars lobbying all over the place to try to prevent people from getting this information. And I think that should make people suspicious. I think it does and it should. I mean, what are they so afraid of? Why are they so afraid to say their technology's out there?

Tamar: Any more?

Patty: Oh, there's so many. I think on that labeling thing, I mean, a parallel industry, a sister industry from biotech is the meat industry. I mean we've been fighting-- again really common, basic information, not extraordinary-- it's been a vicious fight for 15 years to get the country of origin labeling on meat and produce. And right now the meat industry is in a full attack on the concept that they have to say where meat comes from. Because they want to say everything comes from the U.S. if they kill the animal here, and they don't want to disclose that the animal was born in another country, like Canada. They want to say it only matters where it dies, not where it lived. And I mean, they're challenging it at the WTO. They're challenging it in court. I mean constant fights to get something that seems so elementary--that you get on a t-shirt or you get on a CD, or a camera-- you know where that was made. But they don't want us to even know where our food was made, like what country it was made in.

Tamar: So they're bringing animals over from other countries just so they can kill them here?

Patty: Yup

Tamar: By ship?

Patty: Ah, no, usually it's by truck. So it's Canada and Mexico are the two biggest so they can just truck them in. But there are proposals--

Tamar: Picturing them, like, flying in from Guatemala.

Patty: No, they do that with fruit, they do that with frozen fish, but with live animals it's trucks. So it tends to be Canada and Mexico. But it's really interesting. I mean, these are multinational companies now, right? It's not like they're Canadian meat companies. They've largely been taken over by U.S. companies and they shut down slaughter plants in Canada. So you have a lot of cattle still being raised there. But the ranchers don't have great options to sell them. So it's become a source of low-cost cattle and they'll truck them, you know, down to Montana or down to Kansas to kill them in slaughterhouses here. So it's not really benefiting Canadian ranchers either. They used to have better options to sell their animals. So as these companies consolidate, they really change these markets. But they still want us to think we're buying locally, still want us to think we're buying from a company we bought from 20 years ago. And it probably isn't.

Tamar: Why, why do you think that is, that they're trying to hide it from us? What, what really are any of these companies trying to hide? Especially the GMO? Why do they not want us to know?

Patty: I think the companies don't want consumers to think too much about what happens before the store. You know, "How did that food get here?" I think they're very happy to market to us. I mean, I always give this assignment to people if they want to think about it-- like, walk through a typical grocery store and count how many products have "farm" in the name or a picture of a silo and a red pickup truck. It's always red. I don't know why it's always red. You know, and a grassy field. And these are not foods that came from a farm that looked like that. Right? They're probably heavily processed. They're probably from a pretty large conglomerate. That is, doesn't look like the picture on the package. They know what we want. They're not providing it. But they don't want people to make that connection.

Ah, and I think you know, what people are really responding to the local food movement, buying at farmers market, you know, getting closer, that's so popular, because people can get closer to the producer and it scares the hell out of these big food companies. They've noticed. It's way more proportionate than the amount of food that's being sold. It's just the concept that you get this information and you realize, "Oh, that's not what they're doing down the road at the giant grocery store. This is different." And they don't want people thinking about those differences. I think that's why they fight all these labeling ideas.

Patty Lovera is the Assistant Director of Food & Water Watch. She coordinates the food team. (http://foodandwaterwatch.org)

Claire: My name is Claire Hope Cummings. I was a
lawyer in the Carter administration, which is probably
the last time you could actually do public service. So
what happened in 1980 was that Ronald Reagan was
elected. And while he was president, several
Monsanto executives went to the White House and
they said, "We've got this new technology." They
hadn't even developed it yet. But they said, "It's
coming on, and we don't want to be regulated, so let's
just leave enough in place to make it look like it's
regulated. We will submit our studies to you. You
rubber stamp them. Then we can say we've got
studies."

That's sort of what it is. It's all voluntary. The
government only knows what the industry tells it. They
don't do any separate studies. And then, the worst
part is, when a few courageous, independent
scientists have come out with studies on their own,
usually funded by themselves or other groups, not by
the industry, they come up with good, solid provable
information about the environmental or the personal
health effects of this, then the industry goes after
them.

I wrote the book, Uncertain Peril, about the future of
seeds for two reasons. One is, I come from a long line
of plant-loving women and I love the natural world.
And what I really care about mostly is the inherent
integrity of the natural world. So I was really alarmed

to find out that there was this new technology which was mix and matching genes and creating new artificial life forms and that there wasn't any regulation and there wasn't any choice on the part of people for whether or not they consumed it, or lived around it. And so it was both to protect what I loved so much and the natural world, and also to raise the alarm for people to say, "We need to know more about this. We need to be protected. If it is dangerous, we'd like to know." Especially food, which is an intimate thing.

Tamar: How has our food system changed in the past 100 years?

Claire: Actually I really love that question. I think that's-- asking how our food system has changed in the last 100 years is really the answer to what we need to know. Because we all come-- maybe we're just a generation or two away from being farmers. Just take the United States. We were all producers. We grew our own food, or we knew the farmer. When I was growing up that's what we did. We bought our food from various places and producers. And we've now become a nation of consumers. And a very few, handful of corporations have taken over all of the production. So they've not only taken over the production of the food; they've taken over the science. They've taken over the technology and the knowledge. They've taken over the rights to own all these things such as seeds, which are the basis of life. And all these changes have happened actually mostly in the last 50 years. So what's going on now is that we are dependent on these large corporations, multinational corporations, whose only motivation is to make money, to sell us what we need.

You know, it's not just food. It's also how we think, what we learn in the news. Everything's been commoditized and privatized and delivered to us prepackaged. You know. Do we have a choice? That's the question. We've gone from having more control over our lives, and more choices, and more ability to connect with each other, and more ability to connect to the natural world, to this massive disconnection where we're being kind of entertained and fed. And I think if people choose that, maybe that's fine if that's what they want to choose. But I'd like to think that people may not know what's involved. What are the political implications, what are the dietary implications, what are the environmental implications? And for me it's also a moral problem.

Tamar: Can you explain what the genetic modification of food is?

Claire: So the genetic modification of food is actually quite simple. It's called recombinant DNA technology. And that means you're recombining, you take a gene from one species and you take a gene from another species and you recombine them and you create a new organism that has both genes in it. And it's usually done for a specific purpose. They want a gene to be able to produce a certain characteristic. And most people don't know almost everything that genetic modification is used for, can be done with natural breeding. You can have insect resistance. You can have draught tolerance. You can have herbicide resistance. These are the things that most GMOs are

[135]

made for. You can do it with traditional breeding. So why is it that we have these genetically modified organisms in our food and in our farming and all over the place? Patents. Patents are the lifebloods of biotechnology.

The reason is, if you genetically modify it, you can own it. And you can sell it. So if all our research money and all our science is going into these artificial creations, what happens to the things that are in the natural world that were gifts of creation that we could use the same way, freely, and farmers could develop them locally to have these plants that would be useful to people?

Tamar: Can GMO technology be a good thing?

Claire: Is there any good to be had from genetic modification? I've really looked carefully at this. I get this question all the time. And my answer is flat out no. The reason is, we have to go way back to why it was developed. It was developed purposefully for the reasons it's being used, which is to patent life and to control life for certain purposes. If we went back and we looked at recombinant DNA technology and we asked different questions about not just what could we use it for, but what else could we do-- and this is the trick to science.

We have to ask the right questions. So, it's not science. It's technology. And with technology we have to know what our motivations are. So GMO technology has never been used or even developed for anything that's any good. One hundred years from now would we be able to use this for some good? I don't know, because it never has been. Now there have been efforts to, what they call, put a moral gloss. Because you see the GMO industry spends hundreds of millions of dollars advertising that their products are going to feed the world, they're going to cure the sick and they're going to end poverty, and they're going to do all these other good things. Well. Let's disregard those nice beautiful ads with starving children with their bowls of golden rice and let's look at actually what GMOs are actually being used for. They're developed by the chemical industry-- Monsanto, DuPont and Dow--big, huge, chemical companies to use more chemicals. So you get Roundup Ready soybeans, Roundup Ready corn doused with way more chemicals than were being used in even chemical agriculture-- industrial agriculture always uses chemicals. But GMO agriculture uses five times as many or 10 times. I mean, the increase in this use of herbicides is just astronomical.

They're also used to make insecticides. Put the insecticides in the plants-- themselves. So you have to ask yourself, "What possible good would it be for us as human beings or for the microbes in the soil or the fish in the water, or the frogs, what possible good would it do for us to be doused with all these very toxic chemicals?" So that's how GMOs are being used. I leave it to you to decide whether or not any good can come from it.

Tamar: So the FDA, USDA and the EPA-- none of these organizations are really doing the job that we think they're doing?

Claire: The three agencies are the EPA-- they regulate the pesticides, and the FDA-- supposedly they are concerned about the allergies. And that's where actually, that one small area of allergies, they actually still pay attention to whether or not that food is an allergen. But again, you have to understand, it's all self-reporting. So they're not doing any independent testing. And these are new artificial organisms. We don't know their impact immunologically. We don't know what happens in nature, or in our bodies. And these are chemicals-- I want to make this very, very clear.

This is the chemical industry. So while the genetic changes might also create a larger protein and present a problem, you also have, like with GMO sugar, Monsanto went behind the scenes and got an okay with no public involvement for a 5,000 increase in the residue of Roundup on GMO sugar beets.

The USDA is really an arm of the chemical industry at this point. They're not even studying the uses of chemicals or the amounts that are being used-- or how they're recombined. It's a total failure on the part of the federal government to stand between the public health, the common good and the greed of these corporations.

The worst part, the worst part of not having any federal protections in our laws, is that we think they're there. We have this idea that government regulation is going to protect us from greed or corruption or pollution. But it doesn't happen anymore. And it's called industry capture. And what happens is, what's happened since Ronald Reagan was elected, is the industries that are being regulated by government have captured the regulatory system. So the FDA is being run by former Monsanto executives.

The decision that patented life, patented seeds was done as well by Clarence Thomas, who was a former Monsanto lawyer. If you just take the Monsanto intrusion into the federal government, it's a good case study of how we don't have any more independence. We don't have independent science and we don't research. And we don't have independence in the regulatory frame.

Tamar: What about BT/GMO corn?

Claire: This BT corn exudes in its leaves and in its roots and in its core, an insecticide. We have no way of evaluating the impact of that insecticide on humankind. And the industry says, for instance, "Oh it's the same as the BT that organic farm is using." The lies are endless. We could spend all day on just, just, the lies. BT that they use is not the same BT as other-- as you can buy in the grocery store. It's been genetically engineered in a shortened form. And the reason I bring that up is because these genetically engineered forms are the ones, the process of doing that, is where the allergens and where the toxicity can come about.

Tamar: Is there a way the USDA, the FDA, and the EPA is supposed to work? Can you explain that chain a little bit?

Claire: That's a really good question. How would regulation work if it was supposed to work? It would be based on the public interest, not on private, you know, corporations. So we would have independent science and we would learn to ask more questions.

Most of the GMOs are herbicide-resistant GMOs-- and they use glyphosates. Roundup is one of the most popular. But it's no longer being useful because nature finds a way to work around these things. So it's lost its effectiveness. So now they want to use a substance that was part of Agent Orange, a defoliant in Vietnam. So now they've just approved, without any questions about its environmental toxicity, 2,4-D.

So now we have 2,4-D corn being grown. And we were concerned about Roundup. So we should be very concerned about this. Were there questions asked about what would be the impact? The answer's no. The USDA just approves these things and rubber stamps whatever the industry tells them. A good way to look at the regulatory system is not as a chain, but as a patchwork quilt with a lot of holes in it.

Tamar: OK, talk to me about synthetic biology.

Claire: I'm always surprised how few people don't know about genetic modification of food and farming. But there are a lot of people who don't know they're eating these genetically modified organisms. Worse yet, is what's coming down now, which is called synthetic biology. So GMOs are about rearranging the genetic structure of organisms. Synthetic biology is about building whole new ones. So they take all kinds of molecules-- they don't just rearrange them, they make artificial life forms.

Tamar: Other countries label GMOs already.

Claire: Sixty countries in the world label genetically engineered organisms and give people a choice. But not here in the U.S. No, no, we wouldn't want to have choice for consumers. Or we wouldn't want to have public science. I think it's shameful. I think bottom line, we should be ashamed of ourselves. We used to think of ourselves as world leaders, being a force for good in the world. And in this instance, we are not. We are exporting industrial agriculture through the military in all areas of the world.

Tamar: Is there any good news?

Claire: Oh there's lots of good news! Oh my god! Thank you for asking that question. It's all good news. I mean, seriously. These problems that we've been talking about are very important. Okay? And we're attending to them. There are so many good people out there bringing lawsuits, protesting, writing petitions, even doing some of the science that needs to be done, taking the place of the bad guys, okay?

There are a lot of good people. So there's more good people than there are bad guys, by far. There's an amazing local food system growing everywhere. The rise of farmers markets is just one way-- from a few hundred to thousands of farmers markets-- and that with it, the local farmers that feed those markets.

Claire Hope Cummings is an award-winning author, broadcast journalist, and environmental lawyer. Her stories are about connecting people, place and plants and respect for the ancient wisdom of traditional land-based cultures. (http://clairehopecummings.com)

Author of, Uncertain Peril: Genetic Engineering and the Future of Seeds.

Carolyn Dimitri, associate professor and director of Food Studies Ph.D. program, New York University. Interviewed 12/4/14

Tamar: All right. So. Tell me your name and where we are.

Carolyn: I'm Carolyn Dimitri and we are in my office at New York University Department of Nutrition, Food Studies and Public Health.

Tamar: And tell me about the NYU Food Studies program.

Carolyn: The Food Studies program is our master's program. We have maybe, 165 young people, somewhere between the ages of 25 and 50. It's a very interesting and diverse group that are here trying to study how to reform the food system.

And, of course, I just gave you a very biased view. Because all of my classes are on the food system. But I have colleagues that teach classes on food culture, so it's really about food in the city-- why people eat it, how people eat it, the meaning to people, and then how it's produced and the problems that are created in our food system.

Tamar: So how has our food supply changed in the past number of years?

Carolyn: You have to take a very broad look at our food supply to see that. If you go to the late 1800s before we had well-developed transportation networks and refrigeration, we had really a series of regional food systems where, like in New York, all of the food was produced in New Jersey-- that's why New Jersey's called the Garden State-- or the Hudson Valley.

But as technological change occurred, it made it possible for farm production to shift around the country into areas that were better suited to food production. So for example, all of our apples pretty much are grown in Washington State, because the climate in Washington, and the soil, are really suitable for apples. So we started seeing specialization in food production. And that was really made possible because we had people urbanizing-- few people moving off the farm.

And then it was, you could actually ship food across the country. So that is kind of the baseline. So when people talk about returning to local and regionalized food systems, I think to me, I interpret it to going back to a time like that. But what those food systems had-- you could never eat anything out of season. Like the raspberries I just had for lunch, you would never be eating those in December. You wouldn't really have coffee, and you wouldn't have chocolate, and you wouldn't have bananas.

So. I just bring this up to point this out that there are benefits to having this highly integrated, globalized food system that we have now. But along with that, of course, has come some costs. Some of the costs are we have fewer varieties of foods being produced. We have food production specialized in different areas of the country, which, I don't necessarily think is bad, but some people think is not really a good thing.

We have really inexpensive food, and because it's produced very efficiently. We have a lot of chemical inputs and mechanized productions that keep the cost of production very low. And then we have low costs all along the food supply chain. But of course, as a consumer, you might think it's great that you can pay 19 cents for a banana, or I don't know how much a loaf of bread costs, two dollars. But underneath that, you have a bunch of workers on the farm and along the food supply chain that really are paid very poorly for their work.

So, I guess the moral of this sort of-- this little story I'm telling is that you-- we have good things in our food system, but they've come at a price. And sometimes the price is food quality. Sometimes the price is the people who are producing the food. And the price can be environmental quality as well, through the use of pesticides and other chemicals.

Tamar: Well, do you think that it's important for GMOs to be listed on packaging?

Carolyn: I believe every consumer has the right to know if they're eating a GM food. So right now, if you want to avoid GMs, you can buy certified organic products. And I believe in certified organic products for many other reasons, other than just the avoidance of GMs. I mean I think they're better for the environment. But I recognize that not every consumer wants to buy an organic product. So I feel if it has a GM product in it, it should be on the front of that label so consumers can make the choice for themselves.

Tamar: Give me an example.

Carolyn: Pretty much any piece of corn you eat that is not certified organic is GM corn. And so, I think people just argue there's no reason to tell consumers. There's like this kind of paternalistic attitude like, "We believe they're safe, why should we tell you you're eating GM food?"

Tamar: What else would you like to say?

Carolyn: You walk into the grocery store and you see everything there. And it's in a grocery store, a food store. And you just assume it is all food. So if you go into the drug store and you look at all of these over-the-counter supplements-- not supplements but the over-the-counter medications-- they've all been vetted to some degree as, they deliver basically on what they promise. So I feel like, if I go through the grocery store, some things are "food" and some things are like "junk food." And maybe "junk food" shouldn't even have "food" attached to it.

So when my kids were little, they would pick up those, you know, terrible cereal boxes. I'm like, "Okay, if you want those, then you can put those cookies back." Right? To make a point that they are-- that's not a substitute for a bowl of oatmeal, or some eggs, or something with some nutritive value. It's basically junk food. So I think that we should just not let that be sold in the grocery store. I think that there should be, like, special stores that have junky food. Or that basically, I'm arguing for more regulation on our food, with stronger signals about what is healthy and what is not healthy.

The fact is, food marketers can sell whatever they want and call it food as long as it has-- like, there's a definition of food. There's a legal definition. I don't know exactly what it is. One of the lawyers has shown it to me. But it doesn't really talk about the wholesomeness or the healthfulness of the food. I think that our food system has left it up to the consumers to decide for themselves. Like, "Here are your choices. You should have freedom of choice." And the fact is, I think it's a little too unfair. It's basically you're telling the food companies you can put whatever you want in the store; and then people have to sort through, you know, thousands and thousands of products and decide what they should be eating. So you know, "Regulate them," I say.

Tamar: Amen. What are some of the biggest challenges we have now? Could be labeling, food production, or anything?

Carolyn: I mean I think those three are the-- maybe the most pressing one right now is the farm worker-- you know, the farmer and the farm worker. Our farmers are aging. Farm land is really expensive. Who's going to grow our food? Who will be growing our food in 30 years? That's a really important question. I'd say that's probably THE most important policy question right now.

And then the next one I think is, how do we get people to work on our farms? How do we make it so that-- how do we stop marginalizing the farm worker? I mean, I feel like a lot of resources are going into looking at environmental issues. We have a lot of conservation programs. People understand that organic is better. I mean, I'm not sure they really understand why it's better, but like, the organic market exists. And so organic farming is increasing. So the free market has come to solve some of these problems. So I think that's from a food production standpoint.

And then, probably the public health people, though, would argue that it's our human health right? We have too many overweight people with food-related disease or diet-related disease. You know, I mean if you think about it, they're all just gigantic problems. I don't know if it would make sense to just address one of them. I feel like, you know, it's hard to separate out and say, "This is the most important."

But over the long term if we don't have anyone growing our food that could be a very big problem.

Tamar: Do you have any advice to the average person out there buying food and wondering what's really in it?

Carolyn: I think consumers should read every food label that they can. I also think that you should be able to pronounce-- you know, this is the advice everyone gives-- you should be able to pronounce all of the ingredients and you should not eat food with too many ingredients. I think if you can live that way, your health will be so much better.

Carolyn Dimitri is an applied economist who studies food systems and food policy, focusing on how food moves from the farm to the consumer. A common thread throughout her research is the role of governmental and private institutions in facilitating transactions between buyers and sellers, including how food labels transmit unobservable information about product quality to buyers and how policies support farmer income and consumer health.

Dr. Dimitri is widely recognized as the leading U.S. expert in the procurement and marketing of organic food, and has published extensively on the distribution, processing, retailing and consumption of organic food. Since 1998, she has published over 35 papers and reports, and given more than 30 talks, on organic food and agriculture. Her paper "Organic food consumers: What do we really know about them?" received a commendable paper award from the *British Food Journal* in 2013. She was recently interviewed on why consumers should buy organic food for an article featured in *Oprah Magazine*.

Research in progress includes a study of urban agriculture in the United States, asking whether the urban setting is a profitable venture for farmers and why urban farms choose to form as a nonprofit organization. Dr. Dimitri is also exploring the political economies of the National Organic Standards Board, which is the advisory council that was created under the Organic Foods Production Act of 1990, in terms of board composition and board recommendations. She is currently writing a book tentatively titled *The US Food System: Economics and Policy*. Recently completed research examined the effectiveness of nutrition incentives, similar to the Food Insecurity Nutrition Incentives included in the Agricultural Act of 2014, on both actual and perceived consumption of fresh produce of low-income consumers.

Prior to joining the NYU faculty, Dr. Dimitri worked as a research economist at the Economic Research Service of the U.S. Department of Agriculture. She is an Associate Editor of the journal *Renewable Agriculture and Food Systems,* and is a member of the scientific board of the Organic Center. She earned a Ph.D. in Agricultural and Natural Resource Economics from the University of Maryland, College Park, and a B.A. in Economics from SUNY Buffalo.

(http://NYU.EDU)

Recommended reading:
Every book by Michael Pollan

Genetic Roulette, The Documented Health Risks by Jeffrey Smith

Gluten Freedom by Alessio Fasano, M.D.

Healthier Without Wheat by Dr. Stephen Wangen

The Irritable Bowel Syndrome Solution by Dr. Stephen Wangen

Seeds of Deception by Jeffrey Smith

Serve To Win by Novak Djokovic

Uncertain Peril: Genetic Engineering and the Future of Seeds by Claire Hope Cummings

Wheat Belly by William Davis, M.D.

For more information, go to FightingForAllergyFreeFood.com or CaptainPurpleProductions.com

www.ingramcontent.com/pod-product-compliance
Lightning Source LLC
Chambersburg PA
CBHW020441290526
45785CB00002B/963